Environment and Health

GLYNTAFF

A division of Hodder & Stoughton
LONDON   MELBOURNE   AUCKLAND

© 1983 Anthony J. Rowland and Paul Cooper

First published in Great Britain 1983
Reprinted 1985, 1989

British Library Cataloguing in Publication Data

Rowland, A.J.
  Environment and health.
  1. Environmental health
  I. Title   II. Cooper, Paul, 19– –
  363.7   RA 565

  ISBN 0-7131-2855-0

Typeset in 10/11 Press Roman by The Castlefield Press, Northampton.
Printed and bound in Great Britain for Edward Arnold, the
educational, academic and medical publishing division of Hodder and
Stoughton Limited, 41 Bedford Square, London WC1B 3DQ by
Athenaeum Press Ltd, Newcastle upon Tyne.

Preface

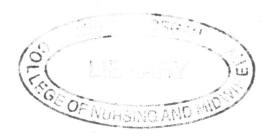

Humans are the end product of a long process of evolution and natural selection — the interaction of biological life forms with their surroundings. The beginning of life itself is still a mystery, but the evidence that has been gleaned suggests that it too originated as the result of interaction of physical and chemical forces. Humans are, in truth, the product of their environment.

Left to itself, life thrives on adaptation, on selection of the most appropriate form, selection associated with the existence of delicate equilibria between organisms and the forces and conditions around them. When changes are not too abrupt, life will adapt and continue efficiently in the new conditions. But evolution is a slow process, and, if changes are too sudden or extreme, then the equilibrium may be upset and life's very existence threatened. Viewed from this standpoint, much ill-health may be seen as the effect of maladaptation.

Humans have doubtless influenced their surroundings on a local scale since they first appeared, but it is only quite recently that human activity has been able to make a significant impact in a global way. They now have immense powers to influence and change their own environment, sometimes in dramatic ways, and have the ability to influence the destiny of all species on earth. Such powers must be used with extreme care. This book sets out to demonstrate how inextricably environment and well-being are interrelated, to examine in detail some ways in which environment and health interact, and to point to the ways in which we may influence both our own lives and those of others for better or worse. The authors are committed to the view that a comprehensive study of the various components which make up the practice of environmental health is necessary to an understanding of its relevance to everyday life now and, perhaps increasingly, in the future. They have attempted to draw these elements together to illustrate how dramatically our welfare and very survival is linked with our surroundings.

The book is written in four parts. The first of these, entitled 'Setting the Scene', examines the definitions of both health and environment and explores some general concepts about the relationships between the two. The second part concentrates on the important health problems which are susceptible to environmental influences, and discusses the evidence which has accrued from epidemiological and other studies, and which points to the environmental causes of ill health. In the third part, some of the important ways in which the relevant environmental influences are measured and assessed are discussed, and the book ends with a single chapter, constituting part IV, in which the various threads of work to improve and safeguard the environment are brought together.

Acknowledgements to the many people who helped in the preparation of this book could run to great length, but special mention must be made of Joy Farrall who prepared the typescript and the owners of copyright material who kindly agreed to its inclusion.

A.J.R.
P.C.

Bristol, 1983

Contents

Acknowledgements

The following tables and figures are reproduced with the permission of the Controller of Her Majesty's Stationary Office: Tables 1.3, 2.5, 2.6, 2.7, 2.8, 4.2, 5.1, 5.2, 5.4, 5.5, 6.1, 6.2, 6.3, 7.1, 7.2, 7.3, 7.5, 7.6, 7.7, 7.10, 7.11, 7.12 and 7.14; Figures 2.1, 2.4, 2.5, 3.9, 4.1, 4.2, 4.4, 4.6, 5.1, 5.2, 5.3, 5.4, 6.1, 6.2, 7.1, 7.3, 7.4, 7.5 and 7.6.

Part I Setting the Scene

1
Health and ill-health

The objective of this book is to explore relationships between the environment in which people live and the health that they enjoy. To be healthy is not just to be free of obvious disease — it is a positive state of physical, social and mental well-being, each of these aspects interrelating with and influencing the others. People who are physically unwell will be anxious, if only a little, about their symptoms; mental distress may evidence itself as so-called 'psychosomatic' symptoms or illness; bad social conditions or social disadvantage bring physical and possibly mental ill-health in their train. Indeed social and behavioural factors are becoming increasingly important as influences on health, so that the social environment is becoming just as important as the physical.

It is important to grasp this concept of positive health from the beginning, for many of us exist in states of less than optimal health without always being aware of it. The occurrence of recognizable disease is, in reality, the last stage of a process which may have been going on for a long time. During that period of unrecognized change, hidden influences have been at work leading to a progressive undermining of the health of the individual. It is important to understand that disease evolves in this way because it may be possible to identify the earlier stages of less than optimal health, so detecting the effects of the environment before they have produced possibly irreversible results. Action can then be taken to arrest the process.

Bothwell (1965) compares the pattern of disease in a community to a spectrum, which not only illustrates the way in which the illness develops with the passage of time, but also demonstrates the various stages which must exist at any given moment within the population (Fig. 1.1). Most diseases pass through its various stages, some more rapidly than others; as in the more familiar spectrum of light, the different parts merge into each other so that there are not sharp demarcation lines as suggested in Fig. 1.1. Different individuals pass through this spectrum from left to right, and through its different stages at different rates. The spectrum illustrates, at one and the same time, how disease as a whole behaves in the community, and how specific diseases behave in individuals.

From the general, or community, point of view, the spectrum can be described as follows. Prenatal life may be affected by environmental influences acting through the mother, adverse circumstances occurring during the pregnancy having harmful effects upon the unborn child. The influences may be severe enough to produce

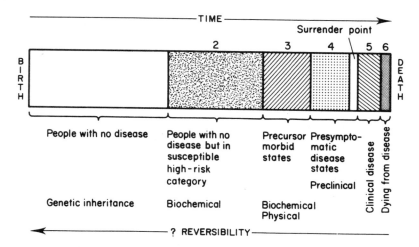

Fig. 1.1   The disease spectrum. See text for details. (Reproduced with permission from Bothwell, 1965.)

imperfection or illness before birth, so that the baby is damaged, or dies in the womb. For example, maternal and foetal infection with the rubella (german measles) virus may lead to congenital abnormality, and the story of how sleeping tablets based on the drug thalidomide resulted in the birth of babies with underdeveloped limbs to women who had taken them during pregnancy is well known.

However, most babies are born healthy, and join the large proportion of the population occupying that part of the spectrum labelled 'people with no disease'. Sooner or later many are exposed to factors in their environment which lead to an increased risk of developing ill-health: this group is symbolized by the second stage of the spectrum. Some such groups are recognizable, as will become apparent in later pages. Obviously, if the environmental hazard to which they are exposed is removed, the deterioration in their health will be prevented, an approach usually described as primary prevention. Those who are in such 'high risk categories' by virtue of their exposure are subjected to subtle interference with the normal functioning of the body, possibly biochemical in nature. In some instances it might be possible to detect some divergence from normal function, but, because of inherent variability, it can be very difficult to assess the significance of such changes. A prime example of this kind of problem can be found in the current debate about the significance of exposure of children to relatively low levels of lead in the environment (see p. 120). Some workers have claimed to detect effects on intellectual development, but the interpretation of the results of the tests and the significance of the findings has been contested in many instances, usually because of imperfections in the tests or technical problems with the statistics.

People in this second stage of the spectrum usually appear to be perfectly well, have no symptoms of any kind, and would not be recognized except for the increasing understanding of the influences of environment on health and the increasing sophistication of tests which can be applied. Eventually, a proportion of these people slide imperceptibly into the third stage of the spectrum. Detectable physical or biochemical changes have occurred and, although they are not yet in any sense 'ill', the early disease process has commenced. Careful examination of such persons reveals bodily changes which are recognizably beyond the margins of normality: for example high blood pressure; unusually elevated blood sugar levels after meals; epithelial cells showing characteristics usually detected in cancer cells, although they do not show any of the abnormalities of cellular reproduction and uncontrolled growth which is the hallmark of established cancer. These individuals have no recognizable symptoms of disease, and would not be identified unless tests were carried out on apparently perfectly well people. This is the theoretical basis of screening programmes in which well people are subjected to tests with the specific intention of finding those affected by such pre-disease states. Clearly, there is no point in doing this unless there is a good chance of preventing further development of the condition, even of putting it into reverse. This type of prevention is known as secondary prevention, and is exemplified by screening for cancer of the cervix (see Chap. 4).

In the absence of any such action, a proportion of those with the pre-disease state develop actual disease, thus entering the next stage of the spectrum. It is not difficult to recognize when this occurs in relatively acute cases, since the onset is fairly sudden and hence noticeable. In many of the slower developing diseases, the early symptoms may not be noticed, or may not be recognized for what they are. The diabetic, for instance, tends to be a little more thirsty than usual, to pass urine more often than usual, and may possibly lose a little weight. As the symptoms become gradually more marked, and perhaps troublesome, the victim decides that something is wrong and seeks medical advice — the 'surrender point'. The stage of recognized ill-health has been reached, but that is a relatively late stage in the total process, and opportunities for prevention have been lost. ('Tertiary prevention' refers to the prevention of further complications, rather than of the disease itself.) Treatment may 'cure' the condition, in which case the patient may well return to an earlier part of the spectrum; but if the disease is progressive, or fails to respond to treatment, the victim enters the final stage.

The maintenance of health largely relies upon understanding, recognizing, and avoiding those factors which are associated with being in the high risk or the pre-disease parts of the spectrum. A large number of these factors have been identified as environmental influences which are often the results of human activity and thus susceptible to human control. Given optimum supplies of nutrients, air, water, space, light and warmth, in an equable social environment, and in the absence of potentially harmful influences, the human organism will thrive. Darwinian theory postulates that it is the environment which determines the optimum organism rather than the reverse, that living creatures have evolved by genetic mutation and the selection, through better survival rates, of those forms of life which are best adapted to the existing conditions. In this way a multitude of life forms, adapted to a variety of different habitats, has evolved. An example of such natural selection is to be found in the case of bacteria where the continuous exposure of an initially sensitive strain to low levels of an antibiotic can eventually lead to the emergence of a resistant strain. The emergent strain possesses a genetic make-up which fits it for life in an environment contaminated by a potentially lethal factor. Similar occurrences have been recognized in the insect world; for instance, the emergence of strains of mosquitos resistant to insecticides has resulted in a serious set-back to attempts to control malaria throughout the world.

There thus seems to be a state of equilibrium between a given life form and its environment. Provided changes are not too abrupt, and sufficient time is allowed in relation to the life cycle and generations of the organism, adaptation will occur. Perhaps, given time, humans could also adapt to environmental change by natural selection, but they are very much more complex organisms than bacteria, and they live and die on a completely different time scale. Starting with a single organism, binary division of bacterial cells once every 20 mins will result in 72 generations and 4.7×10^{21} organisms in one day of a humans' life. By the use of their innate qualities of intelligence, humans can adapt to life in varying conditions, but this is not a genetic adaptation, which would take many generations to become apparent. Thus, if the balance between ourselves and our environment is changed by the introduction of some potentially harmful factor, either by natural occurrences or by human action, then human health and even survival may be affected. In this sense, preservation of health results from maintenance of the natural state of equilibrium, and conversely, ill-health can be viewed as the result of maladaptation to a hostile environment.

It must be recognized that in recent years the Darwinian concept of evolution has been under increasing attack on both religious and scientific grounds. The creationists believe that the creation of the world as described in Genesis is quite literally true; the whole of the existing universe was created in seven miraculous days. Scientific criticisms are based mainly on the failure of palaeontologists to find proof in fossil remains of the unbroken chain of evolution which is predicted by Darwinian hypothesis. It is not the purpose of this book to become embroiled in this argument. Some evolutionary sequences can be traced in fossil remains, such as the evolution of the modern horse from a much smaller animal, and examples have already been given of currently recognized selection of the fittest organisms for a given environment.

Health is a relative state, and a base-line from which to measure health is needed. In theory, this would be the optimum state of the organism. What such a state might be can only be recognized by measuring the characteristics of a large number of people and attempting to identify the appropriate level of each of the characteristics to be taken into account. Several problems emerge. Firstly, it may be difficult to devise a way of actually measuring certain aspects of health, in the sense of fitness, or of social well-being or mental state. Secondly, there is enormous variability in the human race, which stems in part from adaptation to the immediate environment. Such adaptations tend to optimize the performance of the individual in the particular circumstances in which he or she is found. Simple examples might be the muscularity of a manual labourer or the digital dexterity of a professional pianist. The Masai tribe of Africa, well adapted to their nomadic way of life in which they cover long distances at a steady jog-trot, have been described by medical examiners as 'capable of out-performing athletes of Olympic standard'. The 'healthiness' of any person, physical, mental or social, thus has to be judged partly in the light of other inherently variable factors; this makes objective assessment very difficult. Research workers have attempted to devise scales by which health status can be measured in a standardized way, but so far, none has found universal approval or applicability.

Nevertheless, if meaningful attempts are to be made to investigate relationships between health status and environment, some way of measuring the level of health of groups exposed to identifiable factors must be found. Anecdotal evidence relating to a few cases is not suitable because of the variability in the human response to which reference has already been made. Epidemiological studies of differences which can be judged to be statistically meaningful (in the sense that the likelihood of the variation being due to chance is extremely low) in groups of people are required. In the absence of measurable indicators of positive health, research workers are forced to measure the occurrence of negative or ill-health which, however, can allow them to focus down upon the detail of identified statistically significant associations between factors and actual diseases. Such research may then reveal subtle pre-disease states occurring in exposed groups. Initial indicators of 'health' status thus tend to be indicators of disease; in subsequent chapters it will become apparent that in many instances associations between disease incidence and environment have been identified and that a better understanding of the relationship has followed careful investigation of the association. Since frequent reference will be made to statistical indicators of disease incidence, some description of these is necessary.

1.1 Indicators

Information about specific causes of *morbidity* (ill-health) and *mortality* (death) can be collected if suitable arrangements are made. In the United Kingdom, as in many other countries, a considerable amount of information is collected routinely. Death is a definable event, and the cause of mortality might therefore be regarded as a reasonably accurate type of observation to make. Mortality data is collected by all developed and many of the developing countries, and is reasonably complete, at least in the former. In the United Kingdom, collection of mortality information commences with the completion of the statutory death certificate by the general practitioner or hospital doctor, or sometimes by the coroner, in respect of every death. The certificate states the immediate cause of death and the underlying disease, and must be submitted to a Registrar of Births, Marriages, and Deaths, who authorizes disposal of the body after registration of the certificate. The local registrars make returns to the central Office of Population Censuses and Surveys (OPCS). In this way the information can be collated centrally.

Attempts have been made to standardize the certifying procedure by designing a statutory certificate and by introducing, through the World Health Organization, an International Classification of Diseases, Injuries and Causes of Death (ICCD). The classification is revised at ten year intervals and the ninth such revision came into force from January 1979.

The tabulations of information produced by this system in the United Kingdom are regularly published in the OPCS *Monitor* series. Information is presented in various ways so that the numbers of deaths from the various causes are separately identifiable within age and sex groups. Figures are given for successive years so that any trends in mortality which have occurred with the passage of time may be recognized. Figures are also given for various regions of the country so that geographical variations can be identified. Before any meaningful interpretation can be placed on such figures, the numbers of deaths must be related to the sizes of the populations in which they occur. (In this context, the word 'population' is used to describe any group of people.) Hence, mortality is usually expressed as death rates, conventionally stated as the number of deaths which have occurred in a given year for every thousand persons alive at the mid point of the year. Mid-year populations have to be estimated, but once every ten years a census is taken, and this provides more accurate figures on which the next series of estimates can be based. The *crude death rate* may thus be expressed as follows:

$$\text{crude death rate} = \frac{\text{number of deaths in the year}}{\text{estimated mid-year population}} \times 1000$$

Such a rate can be calculated for any specified population − it may be applied to the whole population of a country, or to the populations of its individual towns and cities. It may be calculated for the same population in different years, for particular occupational groups, or separately for the age and sex groups which make up the population; the latter are called *age* and *sex specific death rates*.

The crude death rate of a population is subject to bias due to several factors. The most obvious of these is age structure, since if there is a relatively high proportion of elderly people, the crude death rate will be raised because of the increased number of deaths amongst them. It is also well known that male death rates tend to be higher, age for age, than female rates, so that the sex structure of a population will also be of some importance. Because of such factors, crude death rates cannot be used for direct comparisons; adjustments, known as *standardization*, have to be made in order to compensate for any such bias. The OPCS calculate weighting factors by which crude rates are multiplied in order to make them comparable.

Another commonly used method of standardization is to derive the *standardized mortality ratio* (SMR). The age sex specific rates of a selected population are used as standard rates which are applied to the equivalent age sex groups of each of the populations being compared. In each case it is thus possible to derive the number of deaths which would have occurred in each age sex group of the populations being compared had the standard rates prevailed. The summation of these will give the total of 'expected' deaths within the populations, allowing for differences in their age and sex structures. Now the deaths which have actually occurred may be compared with those expected; the ratio between observed and expected is the standardized mortality ratio, often expressed as a percentage:

$$\text{SMR} = \frac{\text{observed deaths}}{\text{expected deaths}} \times 100$$

The standard population will clearly have a SMR of 100, whereas other populations, compensated for age and sex differences, will have SMRs greater or lesser than 100 depending upon their relative levels of mortality.

A particularly important example of an age specific mortality rate is that of children aged less than one year, the *infant mortality rate*, with a number of subdivisions (Table 1.1). Infant mortality is very sensitive to adverse environmental conditions, and this is particularly the case with the post-neonatal rate. There has been a considerable drop in infant mortality in England and Wales during the twentieth century as general social conditions have improved. In modern times, most infant loss in developed countries occurs during the very early days of life and is associated with immaturity, congenital abnormalities and obstetric difficulties.

There are a number of examples of routinely gathered morbidity information, but all are subject to constraints which restrict their value and often make them unsuitable for use in investigations of environmental effects on health. Sickness benefit claims are related only to the working population. Although the cause of disability is stated on the certificate by the certifying medical practitioner, the of predatory birds. As a result they produced soft-shelled and infertile eggs, and their numbers began to decline dramatically. Had these birds been exterminated, there might have been changes in the populations of rodents which formed their prey.

Humans have evolved as a result of selective processes and consequently are adapted to the environment in which they find themselves. But an important new factor has been introduced as a direct result of their evolution — they have acquired intelligence, knowledge, and expertise which enables them to make significant and dramatic changes to their own environment, changes which are becoming increasingly extensive at an apparently accelerating pace. These have a 'feed-back' effect, and some may lead to conditions less suitable to the human bio-logical constitution. Potentially most dangerous of all are the effects of human activities on the chemical and physical environment which may produce quite dramatic and extreme changes far too rapidly to allow the relatively gentle ad-justments associated with natural selection of biological characteristics to suit the new conditions. It has already been pointed out that these changes may also affect other forms of life, disturb the ecological balance, and ultimately impinge indirectly on human well-being. From this point of view human ill-health may be regarded as a manifestation of inadequate adaptation to environmental change, some of it self induced. Effects vary from the slight, such as anxiety caused by the pressures of a modern high-speed high-technology society, to extreme, such as serious incapacitation or death following exposure to a chemical poison.

The environment has many facets, seen and unseen, real and abstract, and it is important to define and consider them in a little more detail. Table 2.1 is a simp-listic subdivision of the main components within three basic categories — physical, biological and social. In this representation, interrelationships in both the vertical and the horizontal directions may be recognized. Vertically, those above set the

Table 2.1 Basic components of the human environment (see text for details).

		ENVIRONMENT			
PHYSICAL			**SOCIAL**		
Geology			History	Folk lore	Tradition
Geography	Climate		Culture	Religion	
	Atmosphere	**BIOLOGICAL**	Politics	Ethics	
Topography	Water supply		Family structure		
	Hygiene	Mircoorganisms	Education	Occupation	Income
		Vegetation	Diet		
		Animals		Nutrition	
		Other humans	Leisure pursuits		
Industry	Transport		Use of tobacco, alcohol, drugs		
Refuse	Pollution		Standards of living		
	Housing		Prosperity		

constraints for those below. Feedback can occur in the vertical direction, especially within the physical categories. For instance, industrial development will influence the characteristics of the atmosphere. Interactions also take place horizontally between physical and social factors. Thus prosperity (a social factor) affects housing and the level of education may influence hygiene and hence exposure to microorganisms, as well as affecting diet and nutrition.

It is important to recognize that environmental factors rarely act in isolation. Consequently it is not often possible to establish a simple cause and effect relationship between a given factor and some specific effect on health. A number of environmental influences are frequently involved; there is a 'web of causation' — a network of interrelated factors all working synergistically towards the outcome. When discussing environmental influences on health these complex multifactorial relationships must be borne in mind, even though, for clarity and convenience, individual factors may be considered separately.

2.2   Geology and geography

The relationship between the geological structure of a country and the health of its population can be well illustrated in the United Kingdom. The rocks in the south east of the islands are geologically younger than those in the north west. The line of demarcation between older and younger rocks follows the limestone escarpment which stretches in a north easterly direction from near the Devon/Dorset boundary on the south coast, through the Cotswold Hills, to merge some sixty miles north east of Bath into the uplands of Northamptonshire. Further north in Leicestershire it forms the Lincoln edge, stretching from Grantham to the Humber. North of the Humber, the last remnants of the limestone are found in the North Yorkshire Moors (see Fig. 2.1). South east of this limestone ridge the surface consists of chalks and clays, younger sedimentary rocks which lie on top of the oolitic limestone, which is inclined, and so runs deeper as it passes south eastwards. North west of the ridge, the older rocks emerge from beneath the limestone escarpment. Nearer the scarp they are exemplified by the older mountain limestones which are found in the Mendip Hills in Somerset, and in the hills of the peak district and of West Yorkshire. Carboniferous limestone is found in association with the mountain limestone, so giving rise to the coalfields in East Somerset, South Wales and the North Midlands. Similarly, mineral deposits occur in the older rocks so that mining for metal ores has taken place to the west and north of the limestone escarpment. Further northwards again the rocks of West Wales, North West England, and Scotland are predominantly the very old igneous and volcanic rocks, contorted by ancient earth movements and in some parts heavily scarred by glaciation.

Rivers, man-made communications such as roads, railways and canals, tend to pass through gaps between the ranges of hills. River estuaries or natural harbours encourage the development of maritime pursuits, including communications with ports overseas, or leisure pursuits such as sailing. Industry develops where raw materials are either near at hand, or where there are good communications for transportation. The coincidence of metallic ores and coal deposits led naturally to the growth of smelting industries near the sources of these raw materials, or in country well linked to them by good communications. The availability of abundant soft water from the Yorkshire Dales was an important factor in the establishment

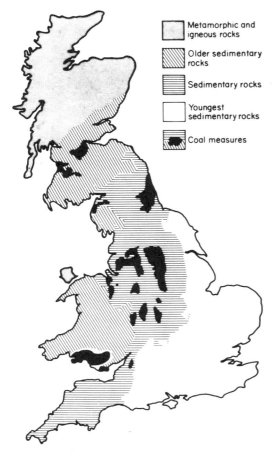

Metamorphic and igneous rocks

Older sedimentary rocks

Sedimentary rocks

Youngest sedimentary rocks

Coal measures

Fig. 2.1 Basic geological configuration of England, Wales and Scotland. (Based on the Ordnance Survey map with the permission of the Controller of Her Majesty's Stationery Office. Crown Copyright reserved.)

of the woollen industry in Yorkshire. Thus the geology and the physical geography of a country affects the occupation and life style of those living upon it.

This division of the British Isles into geological zones, lying in the north west and south east is associated with a gradation of mortality from all causes as measured by standardized mortality ratios (Figs 2.2 and 2.3). The SMRs of local authority districts are found to be lower, generally, in the south east than in the north west. This association between geology and mortality is an indirect association, mediated through the physical and social effects of the distribution of industrial activity and its accompanying urbanization. Geological factors can also have a direct influence on health because of variations in the occurrence of trace elements important to health. The long recognized association of enlargement of the thyroid gland (goitre) with residence in the Derbyshire peak district is related to a local deficiency of the trace element iodine. Variations in fluoride levels are associated with variations in the incidence of dental caries. Hard water supplies derived from limestone areas, with their relatively high levels of calcium and

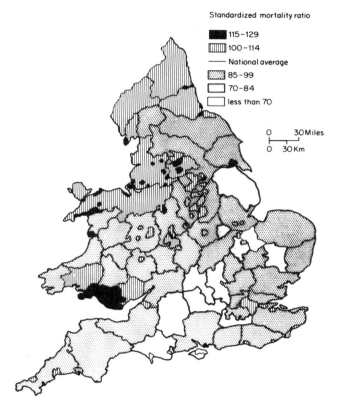

Standardized mortality ratio

- ▮ 115–129
- ▨ 100–114
- — National average
- ▨ 85–99
- ☐ 70–84
- ☐ less than 70

0   30 Miles

0   30 Km

Fig. 2.2   Mortality from all causes — males (U.K.). (Adapted and reproduced with permission from Howe, 1970.)

magnesium appear to be associated with reduced mortality rates from cardiovascular diseases, although the mechanism of this apparent protective effect has not yet been elucidated.

Careful observations of variations in geographical distribution of disease can thus point to the influence of local environmental factors. Observations of the effects of migration to and from places of high prevalence of disease can assist in separating racial and genetic or cultural effects from those of the physical environment. Conditions caused by local environmental factors affect only those living there, the risk of developing them diminish after they leave, whereas, if the factor is genetic the resultant excess incidence is seen in affected persons no matter where they live (see page 55).

2.3   Climate

Climate is of considerable importance to health. The occurrence of communicable diseases may be influenced by the effects of prevailing temperature or humidity on the causative organisms, insect vectors, or infected individuals. Climate influences

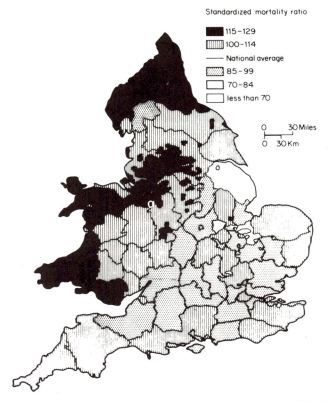

Standardized mortality ratio

- 115–129
- 100–114
- National average
- 85–99
- 70–84
- less than 70

0   30 Miles

0   30 Km

Fig. 2.3   Mortality from all causes – females (U.K.). (Adapted and reproduced with permission from Howe, 1970.)

the conditions under which people live and work, the kinds of housing that they enjoy, and the clothing that they wear. Humans are well able to adapt to life in varying climatic conditions, but instances of maladaptation leading to ill-health can be recognized.

Exposure to sunshine has a direct bearing on health. Vitamin D is synthesized in the skin under the influence of ultraviolet light from the sun. When dark-skinned individuals, adapted to climates where prolonged exposure to the sun is the norm, move to less sunny climates it may become necessary for them to increase their dietary content of Vitamin D. In recent years signs of Vitamin D deficiency, including rickets, have reappeared in Britain, particularly in more northerly latitudes, amongst Asian immigrants. Especially in the more sunny countries, constant exposure to the sun is associated with an increased incidence of the relatively uncommon skin cancer melanoma in fair-skinned races (see Chap. 4).

Heat leads to sweating and associated salt depletion; inadequate dietary replacement of salt can then lead to muscle cramps. A similar sequence may occur if working conditions are accompanied by exposure to abnormally hot temperatures (see Chap. 11). In hot climates sweat glands may become overstressed and eventually fail in those who have not been able to acclimatize adequately. The skin condition known as prickly heat is a manifestation of sweat gland failure. Interference with the control of body temperature caused by sweat gland failure or excessively humid conditions which may prevent the efficient evaporation of water from the surface of the skin can result in heat stroke which may be life threatening.

Extremes of cold are also potentially harmful; they may cause local tissue damage (frost bite) or may lead to a generalized fall in body temperature accompanied by a loss of heat control (hypothermia) — a condition to which the very young and the very old are particularly vulnerable. The effects of exposure to cold air are aggravated in wet conditions, especially if the air is moving, since the evaporation of the water increases the cooling effect. Bad housing is often damp and draughty and thus very cold in the winter months, and these factors doubtless play their part in undermining the health of the occupants.

Human industrial activity leads to atmospheric pollution, and, if the air is relatively still, the resultant accumulation of pollutants may become harmful to health. Such conditions are liable to occur in the atmospheric conditions known to meteorologists as an inversion. In past years in Britain, the combustion of bituminous coal in inefficient domestic fireplaces and factory furnaces resulted in severe atmospheric pollution in urban areas. In inversion conditions, the resulting combination of smoke, sulphur dioxide and other pollutants within a pool of cold stagnant foggy air led to a dirty fog known as smog. These conditions are very harmful and even potentially life threatening to those already suffering from severe respiratory or cardiovascular disease. Repeated exposures of lung tissues result in damage to the delicate lining of alveoli and bronchioles (see Chap. 6).

Anticyclones, once established, are fairly stable and smog conditions may persist for many days, the air becoming increasingly polluted as time goes by. London and other large cities in Britain suffered intermittently from smog conditions over many years, as did locations in other industrial countries. The conditions and their effects became steadily worse as the degree of atmospheric pollution increased, and, in Britain, culminated in the disastrous London smog of 1952, when some 4000 victims were believed to have died as a direct result. The effective reduction of atmospheric pollution in Britain through the implementation of the Clean Air Act, 1956, has been markedly successful in preventing such conditions so that severe smogs of this nature no longer occur.

Photochemical smog results from the interaction of nitrogen oxides from vehicle exhausts with hydrocarbons in the atmosphere under the influence of sunlight. Oxidizing agents are formed, such as ozone and peroxyacetyl nitrate, which irritate the eyes and respiratory passages. This kind of smog is not a troublesome problem in Britain, where the level of ultraviolet radiation from the sun is not prolonged or intense enough to create high concentrations of oxidants, but it has been reported, for instance, in the U.S.A., where Los Angeles in particular is severely affected from time to time.

In parts of the world where rainfall is sparse, or only occurs for part of the year, efficient methods of collecting and conserving water supplies become important, an adequate water supply being important for the preservation of good standards of hygiene as well as for drinking and cooling purposes. Modern methods of sewage disposal rely on water carriage, and where sanitation is inefficient there is an increased risk of the proliferation and transmission of infectious diseases, especially those affecting the gastrointestinal tract.

Climatic conditions also determine the characteristics of other life forms with which the human population must co-exist. Insects, which may act as efficient transmitters of infection, are particularly active in warmer climates. The classical example is the mosquito, certain species of which are specifically related to the transmission of several diseases (Table 2.2). The climatic conditions must be appropriate if mosquitos are to transmit infection — malaria is not transmitted in Britain at the present time (although it has been in the past).

Table 2.2   Diseases transmitted by mosquitos.

Disease	Species
Dengue syndromes	
Onyognyong virus	*Anopheles*
West Nile dengue	*Culex*
Dengue viruses	*Aedes aegypti*
Filiariasis	*Aedes, Anopheles, Culex, Mansonia*
Malaria	*Anopheles*
Virus encephalitides (e.g. equine encephalitis, St Louis encephalitis, Japanese B encephalitis)	*Aedes, Culex*
Yellow fever	
Urban	*Aedes aegypti*
Rural	*Aedes simpsoni, Aedes africanus*

2.4   The living environment

Part of the physical environment is the life around us. The science of ecology describes the dynamic interrelationships between various life forms in a given habitat and the ways in which the well-being or failure of one may well have profound influences on the status of others (see Anderson, 1981). Bacteria break down organic compounds into less complex substances and hence contribute to the recycling of many of the raw materials essential to life. Others synthesize important compounds, for example bacteria in the gut synthesize vitamin K and some of the many substances making up the vitamin B complex, although, in the human, probably only the folic acid so synthesized can be absorbed. In animals such as rodents, where coprophagy (dung-eating) is the norm, other vitamins may be absorbed from the dung. The developing science of genetic engineering is opening up possibilities of utilizing the manufacturing abilities of some bacteria for the production of medicinally important substances. It has been recognized for some time, of course, that microscopic fungi produce antibiotics in the natural course of events, and genetic engineering was not necessary to reap that harvest.

Microorganisms exist around, on, and in us, and for most of the time this co-existence is harmonious even though some of them are capable of invading human tissues and causing harm in appropriate circumstances. This state of equilibrium depends partly upon the maintenance of a dynamic balance between the vigour and invasiveness of the microorganism and the state of the body's defences. If the defences fail an opportunity may be provided for ordinarily inoffensive organisms to cause disease and even to become lethal. Less commonly, the organism itself may undergo a change which enables it to overcome normally adequate defence mechanisms. Sometimes invading organisms are destroyed completely, sometimes a state of equilibrium is regained. Less often the organism prevails, and disease ensues. Every day we have these encounters with the invisible life around us, and, for most of the time, know little of it.

The visible animal life around us is a more apparent, and equally important, part of the environment. Animals contribute to our recreation and their presence gives aesthetic pleasure and so enhances the quality of life. The work role of some animals has become less important because of the advent of machinery, but some are still an important source of food. Animals can also act as reservoirs of infectious disease agents. Thus it is important that wild life should be preserved, that farm and domestic animals are kept in good health, and that whatever possible is done to detect and control the transmission of infectious diseases of animals, including those which can be transmitted to humans (see p. 35).

2.5   The continuing industrial revolution

Factors which are important for the maintenance of a good quality of human life include clean air, a good supply of clean and wholesome water, light, especially sunlight, adequate space for living and recreation, a reasonably equable temperature without extreme changes, a plentiful supply of nutrients free from injurious contamination, access to reasonably quiet and peaceful surroundings in which to take rest, and a congenial relationship with those with whom we come into contact. The human propensity to live in groups heightens the risk of competition for these life factors. Such a system of living is at once both mutually supportive and mutually destructive, and the right balance has to be achieved. One of the destructive factors in the equation is the accumulation of dejecta and rubbish which any group produces. Unless some means of removal and safe disposal evolves, the quality of life inevitably deteriorates through the contamination of air, food, and water, and the general aesthetic despoilation of the environment. When the processes of normal domestic life are added to the results of modern sophisticated industrial technology the hazards of environmental contamination become increasingly significant.

The village economy of the 17th and early 18th century was doubtless imperfect in many ways. However, there was certainly more space in which to live and in which to grow food for the family. The air was relatively clean, and there was a simple way of dealing with the detritus of daily life. The garbage heap and the privy, separated from living quarters, and from the well which was the source of water, provided means of naturally recycling materials. With the advent of factories, and the towns which grew around them, the rural habits of living were transplanted with the people, but in the changed conditions of crowded urban living, the system suddenly failed. Massive accumulations of refuse and excreta, no longer adequately recycled, contaminated yards and streets, water and food, with disease producing organisms. Crowding together of large numbers of dwellings reduced available space and light. The crush of bodies heightened competition and destroyed opportunities for rest. Food supplies became more difficult to obtain, overwork and undernourishment became rife. Heavy bacterial contamination of the environment coupled with overcrowding led to massive outbreaks of infection. The quality of life deteriorated seriously, and the resulting mortality was severe, associated with widespread epidemics of serious infectious disease. The problems were largely those of inadequate disposal of domestic refuse and excreta, inadequate water supplies, bad housing, and overcrowding. Leaders like Edward Chadwick and Sir John Simon emerged to form the vanguard of the attack on these appalling environmental conditions, and, very gradually, matters were brought under control and conditions improved.

McKeown (1979) refers to the considerable fall in death rates which has occurred during the past three centuries and indicates the very considerable part played by the reduction in mortality due to infectious diseases (Table 2.3). There can be little doubt that even in the days before the industrial revolution, infectious disease was an important agent of death, especially amongst children. Nevertheless, history has clearly recorded the cataclysm which was engendered by the shift from village to urban dwelling and which awakened the consciousness of thinking people of the time to the seriously adverse effects which the new environment was having on human health.

Table 2.3 Reduction of mortality since 1700 in England and Wales. (Reproduced, with permission, from McKeown, 1979.)

Period	Percentage of total reduction in each period	Percentage of reduction due to infection
1700 to 1848–54	33	?
1848–54 to 1901	20	92
1901 to 1971	47	73
1700 to 1971	100	

The estimates are based on the assumption that the death rate in 1700 was 30

However, the industrial revolution is not just history — it is still present. Those were the days of domestic pollution, these are the days of industrial pollution, for we are now grappling with the problems of safely controlling and disposing of the materials which spill out of and are thrown away by factories, foundries, refineries, and all the other elements of an industrial nation. At the same time all those other factors which determine the quality of life are directly affected by an industrial environment. The old problems of sanitation have been largely overcome, although there is still concern with the maintenance of adequate standards. The problems are often those of economics rather than of 'know-how'. High rise flats, for instance, are no doubt very efficient in terms of land economy, but they take no real cognisance of the human need for space, light and privacy.

The new problems which have to be faced are those resulting from industrial pollution and the growth of large cities — noise, smoke and other emissions from factory chimneys, effluents, contamination of the environment by escapes or discharges of chemicals, or of radioactive materials, general aesthetic deterioration associated with obsolete machinery, rubbish, dereliction, accumulations such as slag heaps and the like. Chemical materials which can now be manufactured and which do not occur 'naturally' are not always biodegradeable and subject to natural recycling processes, and as a result they may accumulate in the environment. For example freons, used as propellants in aerosol cans, are accumulating in the atmosphere and have given rise to some anxiety because of the theoretical possibility that they may in time interfere with the climate of the world. Some chemicals may have untoward effects on biological systems which have not adapted to them through the normal slow processes of evolution (Duffus, 1980). Massive doses may have obvious and immediate toxic effects, but there is also evidence that smaller quantities of some chemicals, which have no immediately discernable effects on well-being, may nevertheless be harmful if exposure occurs over a prolonged period. Such effects are manifestly more difficult to detect and measure; much modern research is devoted to seeking them out. It is easier to recognize more dangerous materials, and these need to be strictly controlled. It may be essential to develop processes which ensure complete segregation of such materials from humanity, and indeed other life forms.

Those at most disadvantage from these various potentially harmful environmental factors tend to be the relatively unskilled, or the manual or industrial workers and their families, living in areas of considerable industrial development, with all its associated problems. Their incomes may be relatively low, while at the same time they may not make the most effective use of the money available to them. Housing standards may be relatively poor, and their diet may consist of foodstuffs of less than optimum nutritional value. Their style of life is thus considerably influenced by the physical environment in which they live.

2.6   The social environment

Life style is also a reflection of the social environment. Much of the culture of any group of people depends on history, and the traditions handed down by their forebears, but, more immediately, life style and sets of values are affected by influences exerted by family and friends. Dichotomies in traditions, culture, and political and religious beliefs cause social groups to be quite disparate and even incompatible. Territorial boundaries may represent not only spatial, but also conceptual and philosophical separation, and it may be difficult, and even dangerous, to transgress them.

Such separation of social groupings is seen in its most extreme form in separate nations. However, within each nation are analagous social subgroups, each tending to have its own life style, although territorial boundaries are usually much less apparent. These subgroups are characterized by different sets of values, religious, ethical, moral and political, and they have differing approaches to, and views about, such fundamental aspects of living as diet and nutrition, dress, work style, recreational and leisure pursuits, the use of alcohol, tobacco and drugs, sexual behaviour, marriage, family life, the rearing of children, education — indeed all the multitude of elements which make up a way of life. There can be no clear cut conceptual boundaries between such social groups, rather they merge into each other as do the colours of the spectrum. Nevertheless, it is important to make some attempt to define and delineate them, for it is becoming increasingly apparent that much human ill-health is related to living standards and living habits, and behavioural factors are emerging as particularly important in the causation of many of the diseases which are posing threats to health in modern times. The importance of this approach to modern preventive medicine is well illustrated by McKeown (1979).

Various approaches to a classification of social groups might be attempted; none is likely to be perfect, each will measure certain characteristics more than others. Occupation is an important aspect of life with which many other social characteristics are found to be associated. Access to, and attainment in, education or training plays a very important part in choice of occupation; conversely, choice of occupation is often associated with the values attached to different kinds of education and to educational attainment. Parental values are influential in the educational progress of the children of a family and hence their subsequent choice of occupation. Occupation also clearly has a bearing on income. Thus these three related factors — education, occupation, and income — are fundamental. In addition, the occupational groups to which people belong influence their life style in a number of ways. Many trades carry their own particular traditions and sets of ethics and principles, and those who work together are likely to share common interests, life habits, and leisure pursuits. Occupation thus stands out as a key factor when defining social groups.

2.6.1 Social classes and socio-economic groups

The social classes defined by the Registrar General are listed in Table 2.4; this classification has been in use since 1921. Since 1951 a different set of socio-economic groups has been in use (Table 2.5) which further refines the grouping of occupation to take other social factors into account with more precision. This classification is an amalgam of occupation, industry in which employed, and economic position. The intention is that each group should contain people whose social, cultural and recreational standards and behaviour are similar. There are 17 groups; the grouping is distinct from the older social class grouping, and one cannot be derived from the other.

Table 2.4   Social classes defined by the Registrar General.

Social class	Description	Example
I	Professional etc. occupations	Lawyers, physicians
II	Intermediate occupations	Teachers, nurses, managers, farmers
III N	Skilled occupations: non-manual	Clerical workers
III M	Skilled occupations: manual	Engineering craftsmen
IV	Partly skilled occupations	Agricultural workers, machine minders
V	Unskilled occupations	Porters and labourers

The different life styles of the social groups so recognized are matched by noticeable differences in their experience of sickness and health. At the level of mortality, this is expressed in the variations in standardized mortality ratios which may be seen in the decennial publications of the OPCS on occupational mortality. Mortality from all causes shows a gradient increasing from social class I to social class V (Fig. 2.4; Table 2.8). Within this overall trend there are many variations. Most diseases show either a consistent rise in the SMR from class I to class V or a rise restricted to classes IIIN and IIIM. Amongst men, important examples of the former in the decennial report for the period 1970–72 are mortality rates for cancer, bronchitis, and other diseases of the respiratory system, and deaths from violent causes such as accidents, suicide, or homicide. The latter category (classes IIIN and IIIM) includes diseases of the circulatory system, ischaemic heart disease (coronary heart disease) and diseases affecting the digestive system. Women show the opposite trend for cancer, but the same trend for respiratory diseases, and a consistent rise in the SMR for circulatory diseases from class I to class V.

Table 2.5   Socio-economic groups defined by the Registrar General (*General Household Survey*, 1975).

Groups		Description
1	1.1	Employers in industry, commerce, etc. — large establishments
	1.2	Managers in central and local government, industry, commerce, etc. — large establishments
2	2.1 } 2.2 }	As 1.1 and 1.2, but small establishments
3		Professional workers — self employed
4		Professional workers — employees
5	5.1	Ancillary workers and artists
	5.2	Foremen and supervisors; non-manual
6		Junior non-manual
7		Personal service workers
8		Foremen and supervisors; manual
9		Skilled manual workers
10		Semi-skilled manual workers
11		Unskilled manual workers
12		Own account workers (other than professional)
13		Farmers — employees and managers
14		Farmers — own account
15		Agricultural workers
16		Members of armed forces
17		Inadequately described occupations

Infant mortality rates have always been sensitive to socio-economic influences (see Table 2.7), and the differences in the rates between the social classes have persisted over the years even though all the rates have shown a steady improvement.

There is similar evidence of an increased level of sickness amongst some socio-economic groups. Table 2.6 shows the average number of general practitioner consultations per annum made by various socio-economic groups, and the numbers of persons reporting longstanding illness.

Much has been done, by central and local government, to improve physical conditions both at home and at work by the continuous strengthening of legislation, through the introduction and implementation of laws such as the Shops, Offices and Railway Premises Act, 1963, the Health and Safety at Work etc. Act 1974, the Clean Air Acts 1956/68 and the numerous Public Health Acts and the regulations made under them. Standards of housing have shown a steady overall improvement and social welfare benefits have been provided. These, and many other measures have been accompanied by significant improvements in general health, seen particularly in the reductions in incidence of infectious diseases and deficiency diseases. However, damaging influences more closely linked to life style and the diseases which result from them are proving to be more intractable. Education in more healthy ways of life is becoming of key importance, and those social groups which are less amenable to educational influences, either because of a relatively low valuation of education, or because of a lower innate ability to absorb, comprehend, or accept new information, are at a disadvantage.

There may also be a natural resistance to changing familiar ways of life which

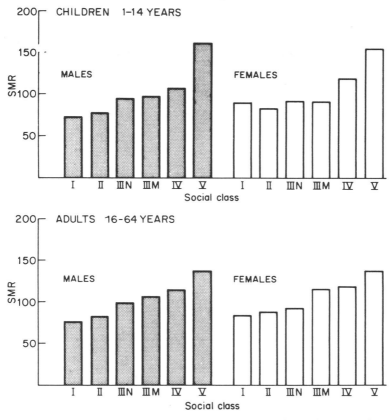

Fig. 2.4   SMRs by social class for all causes of death in England and Wales, 1970–72. (From OPCS, 1978.)

are, perhaps, part of the social culture, and, in some cases, actual difficulty in making such changes because of consequent effects upon bodily comfort and immediate well-being. Perhaps the best example of this kind of problem is the habit of smoking cigarettes, a well ingrained cultural practice with strong social connotations, the cessation of which, in an habituated individual may cause considerable discomfort and malaise. The damaging effects of cigarette smoking are now well documented and publicized. Yet certain social groups in the population have been much less successful than others in reducing their use of cigarettes, and consequently are continuing to pay a price, in terms of morbidity and mortality, which those who have stopped the habit are beginning to escape (see Fig. 2.5).

It has been found repeatedly that members of social classes IV and V are less likely to respond to health education, less likely to attend preventive health clinics such as antenatal, child health or screening clinics, and less likely to take advantage of protective services such as immunization for their children. At the same time, these are the people who are most exposed, at home and at work, to potentially damaging influences in the physical environment. There are thus good reasons why

Table 2.6   Morbidity and socio-economic status (from *General Household Survey*, 1975).

Socio-economic groups (see Table 2.5)	Average GP consultations per person per year		Persons reporting long-standing illness (rates per thousand)	
	Males	Females	Males	Females
Professional (Groups 3, 4)	2.7	3.5	168	149
Employees and managers (Groups 1, 2, 13)	2.7	3.5	216	212
Intermediate and junior non-manual (Groups 5, 6)	3.1	4.2	229	224
Skilled manual and own-account non-professional (Groups 8, 9, 12, 14)	3.0	3.6	227	216
Semi-skilled manual and personal service (Groups 7, 10, 15)	3.5	4.3	268	293
Unskilled manual (Group 11)	3.3	3.8	331	377

Table 2.7   Child mortality by social class, 1970–72, England and Wales (from OPCS, 1978).

Social class	Stillbirth rates		Infant mortality rates		SMRs children 1–14 years	
	Male	Female	Male	Female	Male	Female
I	9	9	14	10	74	89
II	10	10	15	12	79	84
III N	11	12	17	12	95	93
III M	12	13	19	15	98	93
IV	13	13	22	17	112	120
V	17	18	35	27	162	156
Unclassified	19	18	29	22	192	183
Unoccupied	12	12	35	28	12	10

particular efforts need to be made to advise and protect them. Readers are also advised to consult the Black Report, *Inequalities in Health* (Townsend and Davidson, 1982).

Table 2.8 Adult mortality (SMRs) by social class, 1970–72, in England and Wales (from OPCS, 1978). All figures for men and women aged 15–64 years.

	Men	Married women*	Single women
I	77	82	110
II	81	87	79
III N	99	92	92
III M	106	115	108
IV	114	119	114
V	137	135	138
Unclassified	100	39	217
Unoccupied	36	3	67

*Classified by husband's occupation.

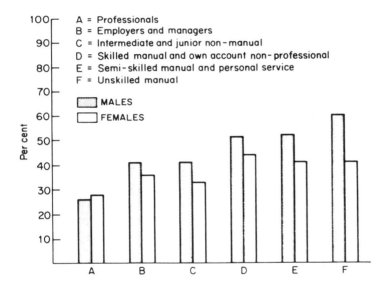

Fig. 2.5 Cigarette smoking status by socio-economic group in Great Britain, 1975. Percentage of each set of groups smoking. (Based on Table 7.33 of the *General Household Survey*, 1975.)

3
Communicable diseases

3.1   The ecology of microbes and man

The agents of communicable disease are microorganisms which are able to live and multiply in other living organisms, in the inanimate environment, or in both. Nature, in this as in all matters, is constantly working towards a state of dynamic equilibrium. The microorganisms are striving to survive, grow, and procreate their own species by reproduction. For this they require appropriate conditions. If a human body happens to be the kind of environment to which the organism is best adapted, the ideal state is that in which both organism and host are able to live and thrive, each without detriment to the other. This is the state of *commensalism.* Even better is a state of *symbiosis*, where the resident organism and its host provide each other with actual benefit. Disease, comprising deviation from the normal physiological state in the host, and possibly the development of environmental conditions inimical to the resident organism, is evidence of disturbance of equilibrium. It may end in the death of the host, the elimination of the microorganism, or to the establishment of a new state of commensalism between the two.

Microorganisms are ubiquitous in nature, and so may be found on or in any material which has not been sterilized. They cannot grow or reproduce, however, unless the conditions are favourable; the most basic requirements are the presence of nutrients, especially protein but also carbohydrates, traces of minerals, the presence of water, and a fairly specific temperature range. They fall into a number of categories — bacteria, viruses, fungi and protozoa.

Bacteria

Until relatively recent times only two major subdivisions of living organisms — plants and animals — have been recognized. Modern biologists consider a third group of organisms — the protista — which are distinguishable as a 'kingdom' in their own right; basically they are the unicellular organisms. The cells of the higher forms of protista are eukaryotic, that is, they have a true nucleus, and have a more complex intracellular structure, with various kinds of organelle. The bacteria and the blue-green algae, classified as prokaryotes, form a separate subdivision of the protista. They have a relatively simple cellular structure, with a recognizable cell wall and a cytoplasmic membrane, but, although nucleic acids are present in the cell giving it a distinct genetic identity, the nucleus is not clearly distinguished as a separate organ. Bacterial cells are very small, their diameters ranging from 10 to 0.2 µm.

Bacteria are primarily classified according to their shape (Fig. 3.1). Cocci are spherical cells; micrococci appear under the microscope as discrete spheres;

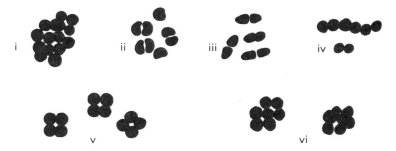

Fig. 3.1 Various morphological types of cocci drawn to approximately the same scale. (i) *Staphylococcus*; (ii) diplococci (e.g. *Neisseria* spp); (iii) diplococci (e.g. *Streptococcus pneumoniae*); (iv) *Streptococcus pyogenes*; (v) micrococci (e.g. *Micrococcus roseus*); (vi) *Sarcine lutea*. (Drawn by A. H. Linton; reproduced with permission from Hawker and Linton, 1979.)

staphylococci occur in clusters like bunches of grapes; streptococci occur in chains like strings of beads; and the diplococci tend to occur in 'chains' of only two. These various arrangements are related to the ways in which the cells divide during binary fission.

Bacilli are rod-shaped cells (Figs 3.2, 3.3). They also occur in varied forms such as plain rods, with or without flagellae; vibrios, which are comma shaped; or spirillae, which assume a corkscrew-like appearance. Some of the more important pathogenic bacteria are listed in Table 3.1.

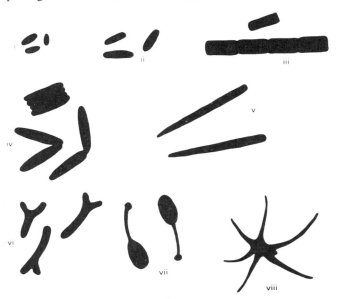

Fig. 3.2 Various morphological types of rod drawn to approximately the same scale. (i) *Serratia marcescens*; (ii) *Escherichia coli*; (iii) *Bacillus anthracis*; (iv) *Corynebacterium*; (v) *Fusobacterium fusiformis*; (vi) *Bifidobacterium*; (vii) *Hyphomicrobium*; (viii) *Ancalomicrobium*. (Drawn by A. H. Linton; reproduced with permission from Hawker and Linton, 1979.)

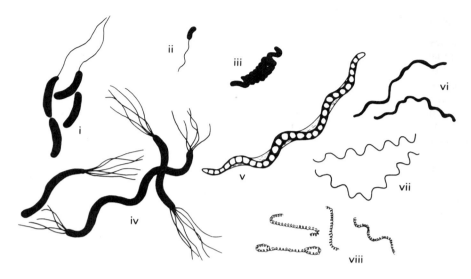

Fig. 3.3   Various morphological types of curved rods drawn to approximately the same scale. (i) *Vibrio cholerae*; (ii) and (iii) *Bdellovibrio*; (iv) *Spirillum*; (v) *Cristispira*; (vi) *Borrelia*; (vii) *Treponema*; (viii) *Leptospira*. (Drawn by A. H. Linton; reproduced with permission from Hawker and Linton, 1979.)

Table 3.1   Bacteria and associated diseases.

COCCI		
Staphylococci		Boils, abscesses, skin infections
Streptococci		Spreading skin infections, sore throats, rheumatic fever, scarlet fever
Diplococci	*Pneumococcus*	Pneumonia
	Gonococcus	Gonorrhoea
BACILLI		
Corynebacteria	(*Corynebacterium diphtheriae*)	Diptheria
Bordetella	(*B. pertussis*)	Whooping cough
Brucella	Br. abortus	Brucellosis
	Br. melitensis	Malta fever
Salmonella	S. typhimurium etc.	Salmonella food poisoning
	S. typhi	Typhoid fever
	S. paratyphi	Paratyphoid fever
Shigella		Bacillary dystenery
Campylobacter	C. jejuni	Infectious diarrhoea
Legionella	L. pneumophila	Pneumonia ('Legionnares disease')
Mycobacteria	*Mycobacterium tuberculosis*	Tuberculosis
Rickettsiae	Various spp.	Typhus
Spirochaetes	*Treponema pallidum*	Syphilis
Vibrios	*Vibrio cholerae*	Cholera

Viruses

Viruses are obligate intracellular parasites consisting of a core of nucleic acid, surrounded by a capsid (shell) of protein, and sometimes further enclosed in an 'envelope' made up of lipids and glycoproteins. Viruses are much smaller than bacteria, ranging from 0.03 μm down to about 20 nm, and contain either RNA or DNA, which in each case may be either single or double stranded. Their nucleic acid content forms the basis of their classification into two main groups (Table 3.2). Viruses are only able to reproduce within living cells; the viral nucleic acid is released from the whole virus and then replicates itself within the cell nucleus. When more viral nucleic acid has been formed in this way, complete new virus particles are built up around it.

Table 3.2 Animal viruses and some associated diseases.

Group	Examples	Diseases caused
RNA VIRUSES		
Myxoviruses	Influenza viruses	Influenza
	Mumps virus	Mumps
Picornaviruses	Polioviruses	Poliomyelitis
	Coxsachie viruses	Virus meningitis
	Rhinoviruses	Common cold
Reoviruses		Possibly diarrhoea in children
Togaviruses	Various arthropod born viruses	Tick borne encephalitis
Coronaviruses		Respiratory tract infections
Rhabdoviruses	Rabies virus	Rabies
Arenaviruses	Viral haemorrhagic fever viruses	Ebola fever
DNA VIRUSES		
Poxviruses	Smallpox virus	Smallpox
	Cowpox virus	Cowpox
Herpesviruses	Cytomegalovirus	Hepatitis in infants
	Simian B virus	'Green monkey disease'
Adenoviruses		Virus pharyngitis
		Corneal ulceration
Papovaviruses		Warts
Parvoviruses		—

Fungi

Fungi are non-vascular plants which lack chlorophyll and have reproductive and vegetative structures which differentiate them from algae and higher plants. They are structurally complex and reproduce either sexually or asexually. Only very few of the tens of thousands of species of fungi cause disease in man. The commonest condition is that of candidiasis caused by the yeast *Candida albicans* — the usual manifestation is a superficial infection of skin or mucous membranes, causing soreness and irritation. Ringworm is also caused by a fungal infection of skin or hair, leading to irritating skin rashes, usually roughly circular, or to areas of hair loss (alopecia).

Protozoa

Protozoa are single celled animals, ranging in size up to about 150–200 μm, although some are as small as bacteria. There are thousands of species, but again comparatively few cause disease in man; examples are given in Table 3.3.

Table 3.3   Examples of pathogenic protozoa.

	Organisms	Disease caused
AMOEBAE	*Entamoeba histolytica*	Amoebīc dysentery
	Acanthamoeba	
	Dientamoeba	Amoebic meningitis (rare)
CILIATA	*Balantidium coli*	Balantidial dysentery
FLAGELLATA	*Giardia lamblia*	Giardial diarrhoea
	Trichomonas vaginalis	Vaginitis (irritation: discharge)
	Trypanosoma sp.	Trypanosomiasis (e.g. sleeping sickness)
	Leishmania sp.	Leishmaniasis
SPOROZOA	*Plasmodium* spp.	Malaria
	Toxoplasma gondii	Toxoplasmosis

Like other life forms, microorganisms are adapted to specific kinds of habitat; many fulfill important roles as part of the web of life. Saprophytes feed on soluble organic compounds derived from dead animals and plants. They produce ecto-enzymes which convert tissues into water soluble substances which are then utilized as nutrients. In this way, saprophytic bacteria and fungi play a vital part in the recycling of the elements needed by living organisms. Saprophytic organisms are often found in the soil and some grow best in anaerobic conditions. Commensal organisms live harmlessly on living hosts, parasites live on living material and cause some damage but not necessarily disease, pathogenic organisms however, cause actual disease. Those which are pathogenic to warm blooded animals are, not surprisingly, adapted for optimal growth at a temperature near 37°C.

Some organisms are adapted to growth in particular body tissues. The rabies virus, for example, localizes and propagates itself in nervous tissue; the typhoid bacillus (*Salmonella typhi*) has a predilection for lymphoid tissue in the walls of the small intestine and for the biliary system of the liver. The gonococcus tends to grow on the mucous membrane lining the urethra, streptococci grow well in the throat, staphylococci colonize the skin. Table 3.4 identifies some of the most common associations between microorganisms and specific body sites.

Figure 3.4 illustrates, in a schematic way, how the surfaces of intestine, lung, or bladder are capable of coming into contact with external materials, as in the skin, whereas the viscera and the blood stream are completely internal and cannot make direct contact with the external environment under normal circumstances. Thus, since the blood is entirely internal only those organisms which depend upon penetration of skin or mucous membrane are likely to be present in it as primary pathogens. Certain bacterial or viral diseases may enter a septicaemic phase in which the microorganism is widely disseminated throughout the blood. This is often a

Table 3.4 Common associations between microorganisms and specific body sites.

Body site	Microorganism
Throat and nasopharynx	Streptococci, staphylococci, pneumococci, meningococci, *Haemophilus* spp., diptheria bacilli
Respiratory tract	Pneumococci, *Haemophilus* spp., *Mycobacterium tuberculosis*
Gastrointenstinal tract	*Escherichia coli, Streptococcus faecalis*, enteroviruses (e.g. poliovirus), hepatitis virus A, *Candida albicans, Shigella* spp., *Salmonella* spp., *Clostridium perfringens*, rotaviruses
Urinary tract	*Escherichia coli, Pseudomonas* spp., gonococci Leptospirae
Skin and hair	Staphylococci, streptococci, *Trichophyton* spp., *Microsporon* spp., *Sarcoptes scabeii*
Blood	*Plasmodium* spp., *Leischmania* spp., hepatitis virus B

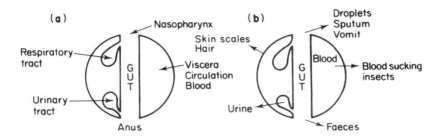

Fig. 3.4 The human body as a source of infection. (**a**) Schematic representation of the body. The body may be regarded as having a tube — the gastro-intestinal tract — passing right through it. In this sense, the lining of the gastro-intestinal tract, as well as that of 'cul-de-sacs' such as the respiratory and urinary tracts, are external surfaces from which organisms can be shed directly into the environment. The viscera and blood, on the contrary, are internal. (**b**) Shedding of organisms from the body.

transient stage in the natural history of an infectious disease, but usually comes under control as the infection becomes localized into its specific site in the body. However, septicaemia may result from the extension and dissemination of a previously localized infection, before the onslaught of which the body's defences are crumbling. This is much more serious and may prove fatal as sometimes happens when such a septicaemia is caused by staphylococci or meningococci.

Other agents of communicable disease

Microorganisms are not the only organisms responsible for human communicable disease. Larger life forms, which may be visible to the unaided human eye, are also capable of living on or in the human body. Most of these are parasites such as the parastitic worms, mites, and certain insects, particularly lice and fleas. Others, such as bed bugs, feed on man but do not live on him.

Parasitic worms are, in the main, bowel parasites, although the guinea worm (*Dracunculus medinensis*) is found in subcutaneous tissues and larva migrans (see p. 38) may occur in various tissues of the body. The nematodes causing filariasis and associated elephantiasis may be found in lymphatics and tissues all over the body; the liver fluke is a resident of the bile ducts. Perhaps the commonest of the intestinal parastic worms is the thread worm or pin worm (*Oxyuris vermicularis*). To the naked eye the worm appears like small pieces of white cotton about half a centimetre long and is almost ubiquitous amongst children of day nursery and infant school age in the U.K., its incidence varying from 20% of children at home to 65% of those in institutions. The adult female worm deposits her eggs, at the anus, and the resulting irritation, which commonly occurs at night, inevitably leads to scratching. The worm may well be destroyed, but the sticky eggs adhere to the fingers and under the finger nails of the child. Children readily reinfest themselves by conveying eggs back to their own mouths, but some of the eggs will be transferred to furnishings and items such as pencils or eating utensils and ultimately find their way to the mouths of others. Fortunately this parasite causes little physical harm to those that it inhabits. Other parasitic worms, such as the tapeworms, or the roundworm *Ascaris lumbriocoides*, which looks like a smooth white earthworm, are uncommon in developed countries, since they depend for their transmission on inappropriate disposal of human faeces or on the inadequate cooking and subsequent consumption of infested meat.

Most human infections with insects are relatively uncommon in the United Kingdom, the exception is infestation with head lice (Fig. 3.5d). Few schools have escaped the experience of discovering head lice amongst their pupils, and this infestation is surprisingly common in our modern and apparently hygienic society. In a study carried out in the late 1960s, nearly 10% of the girls and 4% of the boys entering school had evidence of infestation, and in another study carried out in the 1970s, 12% of children returning to school at the end of the summer holiday were infested. The persistence of head lice is facilitated by the fact that they live on the hair and attach their egg cases firmly to it, so that they are not eliminated by ordinary washing. Body lice (Fig. 3.5b) and fleas (Fig. 3.5a), on the other hand, live in the seams of clothing, and are found on the skin only when feeding. Adequate changing of clothing, associated with proper laundering, therefore disposes of these infestations; they tend to occur in conditions of extreme squalor where personal cleanliness is virtually non-existent. Occasionally, a small infestation may occur in cleaner surroundings, but, for the reasons stated, does not survive for long.

There is, however, a relatively common mite, *Sarcoptes scabiei* (Fig. 3.5e) which lives actually in the epidermis, and causes the skin condition known as scabies. The infestation is transferred by the migration of a gravid female mite from one person to another, and usually depends upon fairly close bodily contact. The mites are not easily transferred through shared clothing or bedding unless the sharing individuals pass the shared materials directly from one to the other, since the mite cannot survive for long away from the human epidermis. In the early stages of the infestation the affected individual is symptom free and, for the first two or three weeks of the infestation may be an unwitting source of infestation to others. In time, however, allergy to the proteins of the mites' bodies and excretions causes the typical rash, and treatment is then sought. This initial asymptomatic period is most important in relation to the spread of the infestation, and must be taken into account when measures to eradicate it are undertaken.

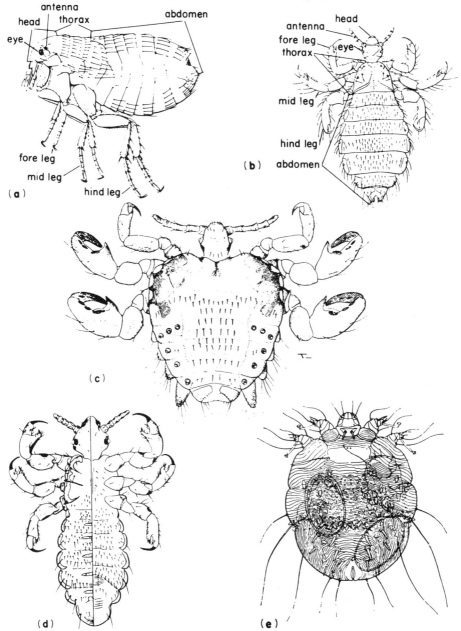

Fig. 3.5 Insects which infest man. (a) Human flea (*Pulex irritans*); (b) body louse (*Pediculus humanus* var. *corporis*); (c) pubic louse (*Phthirus pubis*); (d) head louse (*Pediculus humanus* var. *capitis*); (e) itch mite (*Sarcoptes scabiei*). ((c) From Smart, (d) after Ferris, both from Smith, G. V. (ed.) (1973). *Insects and other Arthropods of Medical Importance*. Reproduced with the permission of the Trustees of the British Museum.)

It is not difficult to understand why the three commonest infestations described above, head lice, thread worms, and scabies, all tend to be family infestations so that it is usually necessary to treat everybody in the family at the same time, whether they have symptoms or not, in order to ensure that the infestation is completely eradicated. It may also be necessary to treat close friends, and possibly even their families. It is usually the failure to observe these cardinal rules which allows the infestations to persist.

3.2   Reservoirs of infection

Pathogenic organisms may be harboured in the animate environment — man or other animals — or in the inanimate environment in materials such as soil, dust, air, water or in contaminated objects or food materials (Fig. 3.6).

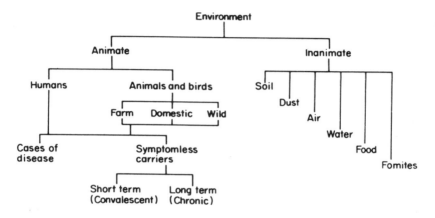

Fig. 3.6   Reservoirs of infection.

3.2.1   The human reservoir

Many diseases which infect humans occur only in humans, and a few of these occur only as overt symptomatic cases, for example measles, mumps, influenza and the common cold. In such diseases, only actual cases are sources of infection; it follows that they must be highly infectious if they are to persist. These diseases are often at their most infectious in the very early stages before the individual develops severe symptoms. But provided that those at risk of developing symptoms can be identified, and all contact between them and susceptible persons can be prevented, then the chain of transmission can be broken. If this can be done with total success for a long enough period of time, the disease can be eliminated, for example as in the case of smallpox (see p. 48).

Many infections, however, move into a state of convalescent carriage, when the symptoms disappear and the victim is well again, but the infection persists and the organism continues to be shed from the body. Such individuals are indistinguishable as continuing sources of infection unless they are bacteriologically, virologically, or parasitologically screened. Temporary (convalescent) carrier states often supervene after gastrointestinal infections such as dysentery or salmonellosis, and carriage may persist for weeks or even months.

Persistent, long term or chronic carriers may have suffered from a recognizable incident of infection at some time in the past, for example carriers of enteric organisms such as *Salmonella typhi*, or may have no history of any significant symptoms. They are often discovered incidentally during the course of investigations for the source of a new case, or because a specimen of faeces is taken for examination for some other reason. Persons who are known to have become chronic carriers following a recognized incident of infection are advised about this fact and of any precautions which may be appropriate to ensure that they do not pose a hazard to others; for instance carriers of gastro-intestinal infections must not work as food handlers.

As the incidence of an infectious disease diminishes in a community, perhaps as a result of specific control measures such as the institution of a programme of immunization against it, the incidence of symptomless carriers does likewise. Although the absence of a carrier state in relation to a given disease means that it is capable of eradication, this is not possible where carriers are able to exist. Thus total elimination of diphtheria is not likely to be achieved, and it would almost certainly reappear in the United Kingdom if the current reasonably high levels of childhood immunization were no longer maintained. There is a constant danger of a 'negative feedback' effect occurring in such circumstances. The continued absence of the disease leads to complacency, mothers no longer worry about having their children immunized, the proportion of protected children drops below the critical level, and the disease reappears. Only by continued vigilance and reminders can this risk be reduced.

3.2.2   The animal reservoir

There are a number of infectious diseases which occur primarily in animals but which may, given the appropriate circumstances, be transmitted to man (Table 3.5). These diseases are known collectively as *zoonoses*. They also may occur in animals only as symptomatic cases, or may be present in symptom free cases as instances of convalescent or chronic carriage. Animal sources can be considered in the three main categories of farm (food) animals, domestic pets, and wild animals. The first two categories, especially the second, are more easily sources of human infection because of their closer association with humans. Persons working with farm animals, i.e. farmers and veterinary surgeons, may be exposed to infections as occupational hazards. Skin lesions such as those of cowpox from cattle, orf from sheep, or animal ringworm, can occur as the result of direct contagion. Veterinary surgeons are at risk of infection by the organism *Brucella abortus*, which causes contagious abortion in cattle and causes a chronic relapsing febrile (feverish) illness of variable severity in humans. Farm animals may also transmit infection to humans through the food chain. An important potential vehicle is milk, which, being a protein-containing liquid, is a very efficient transport medium for bacteria. Bovine tuberculosis and brucellosis can be transmitted to consumers. There have also been outbreaks of paratyphoid fever, spread from cattle through milk, although in these cases the cattle were originally themselves infected from a human source contaminating the stream from which they drank.

Pasteurization of milk is an important measure which blocks such transmission of infection from farm animals. Steps have also been taken to eradicate both tuberculosis and brucellosis from cattle. The former has been virtually totally eradicated for many years, brucellosis has been eradicated more recently. The campaign

Table 3.5   Animal reservoirs of infection.

Disease	Organism	Transmission	Reservoirs
VIRUSES			
Equine encephalitis	Various	Tick bites	Birds, rodents, horses
'Green monkey disease'	Simian B virus	Direct (bites)	Monkeys
Cat scratch fever	Cat scratch virus	Direct (scratches)	Cats
Cowpox	Cowpox virus	Direct contact	Cows
Orf	Orf virus	Direct contact	Sheep
Psittacosis	Psittacosis virus	Dust, droplets	Psittacine birds (e.g. parrots, budgerigars), pigeons, poultry
Rabies	Rabies virus	Direct (bites)	Canines, felines, bats
RICKETTSIAE			
Typhus	*Rickettsia typhi, R. australis, R. tsutsungamushi,* etc.	Tick bites	Various rodents
Q-fever	*Coxiella burnetii*	Dust, droplets, milk	Cattle, sheep, goats
BACTERIA			
Anthrax	B. Anthracis	Contact with blood (wet or dry)	Ruminants
Brucellosis	*Brucella abortus, Br. melitensis*	Contact (droplets), milk	Cattle, goats, pigs
Erysipeloid	*Erysipelothrix*	Contact (carcase)	Pigs, poultry, fish
Leptospirosis	*Leptospira* sp.	Water contaminated with animal urine	Canines, rodents, pigs and cattle
Plague	*Pasteurella pestis*	Flea bites	Rodents
Salmonellosis	*Salmonella* sp.	Faeces, carcase meat	Cattle, sheep, pigs poultry
Tuberculosis	Mycobacteria	Contact (droplets), milk	Cattle, goats, pigs, cats, dogs
FUNGI			
Ringworm	*Microsporon* sp., *Trichophyton* sp.	Direct contact	Dogs, cats, horses, cattle, poultry
PROTOZOA			
Leishmaniasis	*Leishmania* sp.		Dogs, cats, rodents
Toxoplasmosis	*Toxoplasma gondii*	Contact (?faecal)	Mammals, birds
Trypanosomiasis, e.g. African sleeping sickness, Chagas disease	*Trypanosoma* spp.	Insect bites	Wild and domestic ruminants

continued

Table 3.5 *continued*

Disease	Organism	Transmission	Reservoirs
HELMINTHS			
Bilharzia	*Schistosoma* sp.	Infected aquatic snails (intermediate host) infect water	Dogs, cats, cattle wild ruminants, pigs
Liver fluke	*Fasciola hepatica*	Contaminated water and plants (e.g. cress)	Cattle, sheep
Hydatid disease	*Echinococcus granulosus*	Faecal contamination	Dogs, cattle, pigs
Tape worms	*Taenia* sp.	Carcase meat	Cattle, pigs
Visceral larva migrans	*Toxocara canis*, *T. cati*	Faecal contamination	Dogs and cats
Trichinosis	*Trichinella spiralis*	Carcase meat	Pigs, rodents, carnivores

started in 1967 and by the end of 1979 only 10% of herds in England and Wales were not accredited brucellosis free. On November 1st 1981 the whole of Britain was declared an attested area; less than 0.3% of herds then remained in the process of qualifying for accreditation.

Salmonella infections may be transmitted through meat. Both cattle and poultry are prone to infection with these bacilli, of which there are literally hundreds of strains. Cross infection between herds, especially of young animals, is common and animal feeding stuffs may also be infected with salmonellae. The carrier state is very common and this makes salmonellosis in animals virtually impossible to eradicate and difficult to control. A small proportion of carcases is always infected so that an important safeguard against human infection is careful food hygiene. Careful storage and refrigeration of uncooked meat will reduce the risks of spread and growth of the organisms until the meat is cooked, when it is sterilized. It is most important, of course, that adequate heat penetration is achieved for a sufficient length of time (see p. 43). Outbreaks of human salmonellosis are almost invariably traced to a breakdown in food handling hygiene. The result in the human is an infective enteritis, with fever, abdominal pain and diarrhoea, frequently followed by a temporary carrier state.

Domestic animals are a potential source of infection, because of their proximity to their human owners, but fortunately are rarely a serious threat since they are less likely to develop a serious illness without this becoming apparent very quickly. It is thus the more occult infections, mainly parasites, which pose hazards in this case. It is very important that young domestic animals are regularly treated with 'worming' medicines even if they appear to be well. Considerable anxiety has been caused by the dog roundworm *Toxocara canis*. The ova of this helminth are deposited with the faeces of the animal. If inadvertently picked up on the fingers, from the fur of an animal or from the grass or soil of a park, and subsequently swallowed, the larvae hatch out in the human intestine. Professor A. J. Woodruff has demonstrated that these ova can easily be found in the soil of urban parks. In the dog the roundworm larvae undergo a complex migration through the blood stream and body tissues, eventually returning to the intestine where they mature and produce fresh ova, so starting the cycle again. In the human, the larvae attempt the same migration, but become, as it were, 'lost', arriving and eventually dying in tissues in various parts of the body as the so-called 'larva migrans'. Although larva migrans are very small, if embedded in a vital organ they may cause serious harm. For instance larva in the retina of the eye produce a granuloma which may mimic the serious malignant growth known as a retinoblastoma, especially in children, causing severe impairment of sight on the affected side and in some cases leading to the loss of the eye.

Ectoparasites (e.g. cat or dog fleas) occasionally bite humans, although they normally prefer life on the species to which they are adapted. Nevertheless, infestations of cat fleas, which have become more common in recent years, can be unpleasant to contend with, since the fleas may be found in large numbers in carpets and furnishings where the cats lie. The rat flea is notorious as a potential vector of bubonic plague. In humans, bubonic plague leads to infection and swelling of lymph nodes, usually with progression to a septicaemic phase which often ends in death. The septicaemia may also lead to the development of plague pneumonia. The victim is then directly infectious to other humans through the medium of droplet borne transmission (see p. 41), and a human epidemic of pneumonic plague may result. The usual sequence of events is an outbreak of plague (an 'epizootic') amongst the rats in a locality, with a consequent increase in mortality. Hungry and infected fleas migrate from the corpses of the dead rats, and may well bite humans, so transmitting the infection to human victims. Thus an outbreak which starts as a zoonosis and an epizootic can become transformed into a human epidemic of considerable proportions, such as the terrible outbreak of the 'black death' which afflicted London in 1349. In modern times, plague is a rare infection of humans, found mainly in under developed countries, or in those countries where war has seriously disrupted sanitation and hygiene. Rodent control, and the recognition of unusual mortality amongst the local rat population, are important in the control of the infection. Vigilance against the risk of importing infected rats must be maintained at sea-ports; the effective control of rodent infestations on ships is a very important part of routine port health measures.

Wild animals, because of the rarity of direct contact with humanity, are mainly reservoirs of insect transmitted infections, whether walking insects (e.g. ticks and mites), jumping (e.g. fleas), or flying (e.g. flies and mosquitos). There are few problems of this kind in the U.K. The virus disease rabies is transmitted to humans by infected saliva, usually as a result of an animal bite. This highly dangerous infection is present, mainly in carnivorous wild animals, in most countries of the world. The U.K. is, however, fortunate enough to be free of it. In recent years rabies has become more widespread amongst foxes on the European continent and has moved from Germany across France. Infected foxes have been found well west of Paris, so that the infection is now within a few hundred miles of England (Fig. 3.7). It is not very likely, although by no means inconceivable, that a rabid wild animal will bite a human. A more likely route of human infection is via an infected domestic animal which has been bitten by a wild animal. Effective rabies vaccines have been developed which will protect even after a bite has been inflicted, but should the victim be unfortunate enough to develop the disease, the outcome is invariably fatal.

Considerable precautions are therefore taken to try to prevent the importation of rabies, which has a long incubation period, into the country. All imported susceptible animals are kept in compulsory quarantine for six months so that if they develop the disease — as some do — they do so in isolation and the risk of further

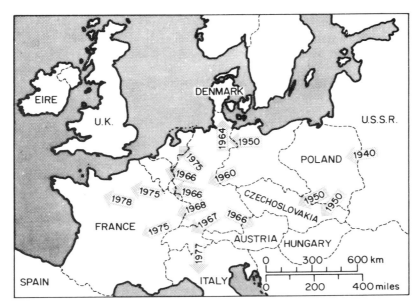

Fig. 3.7   The spread of rabies in Europe, 1940–79. (Reproduced with permission from MacDonald, D. W. (1980). *Rabies and Wildlife*. Oxford University Press. ©Earth Resources Limited, 1980.)

spread is nullified. There is always a risk that some misguided person will attempt to circumvent these precautions and smuggle an animal into the country. Heavy penalties may be imposed on those caught in this particular act.

3.2.3   The inanimate environment

Soil organisms which may cause human disease are the anaerobic spore bearing clostridia. Clostridia are also found as commensals in the faeces of animals; they all grow best in anaerobic conditions such as those associated with necrotic body tissue or foreign bodies impacted within wounds. Gas gangrene (*Clostridium perfringens*) and tetanus (*Cl. tetani*) are both infections which may occur following contamination of wounds with infected soil. *Cl. botulinum*, the cause of botulism, may contaminate inadequately bottled vegetables or fruit and has been found in imperfectly canned tinned meats, fish pastes and pâtés where there is a low oxygen tension and dead organic material. The slow growth of the organism in these conditions contaminates the food with its very dangerous exotoxin (see p. 46), which, when consumed with the food has serious effects upon the nervous system.

Pathogenic organisms found in dust are derived from detritus or discharges from infected persons. Hair, skin scales, droplet nuclei, crusts and sloughs from lesions, and traces of dried faeces are among the potential sources. Inanimate objects (fomites) may be contaminated. John Snow recorded how, during the cholera epidemic of 1832 a package of clothing formerly belonging to a victim of the cholera in Leeds was sent to the village of Moor Monkton in Yorkshire, where it initiated a disastrous outbreak of cholera amongst the local inhabitants.

Food and drink may become accidentally infected by dust, contaminated utensils, infected fingers, or by animals or insects (e.g. rodents, birds, cockroaches) gaining access to it. Meat, as we have already seen, may be contaminated with salmonellae at source. Water is open to contamination in areas from which it is collected, potential sources being animal or human excreta, and so requires cleansing and sterilization before it is used for drinking purposes (see Chap. 7). Stagnant water may also contain organisms such as amoebae, fungi or bacteria. This may be of importance when the water is used repeatedly in cooling towers or humidifiers which form part of air conditioning systems. The condition known as 'humidifier fever' which affects staff working in air conditioned premises, is believed to be an allergic response to materials derived from such organisms present in the humidifier water. More serious have been the occasional outbreaks of the so-called Legionnaires disease. This was named after the first recognized outbreak following a convention of Legionnaires (American ex-servicemen) in Philadelphia, U.S.A., in 1976. The cause was identified as a bacterium which has been appropriately named *Legionella pneumophila*, and which, although previously unrecognized, is frequently present in water, growing in water kept above 20°C. If such heavily contaminated water is used in air conditioning systems the living microorganisms can be dispersed as an aerosol through the system; the air in the building becomes heavily infected, resulting in the occurrence of a pneumonia in susceptible persons. This is a very recent instance of how, by changing their own environment, humans may upset the ecological balance, and so lead to an entirely new health problem.

3.3   Transmission of infection

For further propagation of communicable disease to occur organisms have to be transferred from a source to a new susceptible individual. Environmental conditions play a very important part in determining the success or otherwise of a pathogenic organism in accomplishing this transfer. The basic modes of transmission are summarized in Table 3.6.

Table 3.6   Modes of transmission of infection.

(1) Direct	By actual bodily contact between infected and susceptible individuals	
(2) Indirect	*(a)*	By droplets or droplet nuclei
	(b)	By the faecal-oral route
	(c)	By contamination of food
	(d)	By 'mechanical' transfer, e.g. by insects
	(e)	By insect bites or invasive medical or quasi-medical procedures such as injections, ear piercing, or tattooing
(3) From the inanimate environment	*(a)*	From infected dust or soil
	(b)	From infected objects (fomites), e.g. clothing, cooking utensils

3.3.1   Direct bodily contact

Comparatively few conditions rely entirely upon direct body contact to effect transmission; they may be regarded as the truly contagious diseases. Venereal infections such as syphilis and gonorrhoea are dependent upon close contact since the organisms (*Treponema pallidum* and the gonococcus *Neisseria gonorrhoeae*) are very delicate and incapable of effective survival away from the body. The same applies, to a slightly lesser extent, to the mite *Sarcoptes scabiei* (p. 32), which again is a poor survivor away from a warm human body and effectively has to walk from one host on to another. Other insect infestations such as lice and fleas may also be transmitted most effectively by close contact but do not rely exclusively on it. Skin conditions such as staphylococcal infections (e.g. impetigo) or ringworm are also transmitted by direct contact, but in these cases indirect contact may also suffice.

3.2.2 Indirect transmission

Droplets and droplet nuclei

Pathogenic organisms present in the nasopharynx or respiratory tract are shed into the environment when disseminated in salivary droplets during the processes of coughing and sneezing, and during speaking. The size of the expelled droplets varies greatly according to the circumstances. A heavy uncontrolled sneeze may project easily visible droplets which soon fall to the ground, as well as smaller droplets which stay airborne for longer periods of time. Small droplets are produced during speech, when saying words like 'tea' or 'four'. If they are very small (say less than 0.1 mm diameter) the droplets may stay airborne, but rapidly evaporate, leaving small particles of solid material which can remain suspended for hours and travel considerable distances. Droplet transmission is one of the most efficient ways of spreading infection. This is well demonstrated by the ease and rapidity with which diseases like influenza, the common cold, measles, chicken pox and whooping cough are transmitted in susceptible communities.

The creation of aerosols by splashing or spraying of infectious liquids in microbiological laboratories can pose a very dangerous hazard to laboratory workers. Reference was made earlier in this chapter (p. 40) to the way in which Legionnaires disease is caused by the formation of infected aerosols in air conditioning systems.

Infected droplets or droplet nuclei usually enter the new host by inhalation, (i.e. through the respiratory tract) although some may be ingested. They may also lead to the infection of fomites, resulting in contamination of fingers and secondary ingestion.

The faecal-oral route

Organisms causing gastrointestinal infections are shed in the faeces. Bad hygiene following defaecation, or inappropriate disposal of infected faecal material can lead to the escape of the pathogen into the environment and subsequent transmission into another gastrointestinal tract. Fingers are easily contaminated following defaecation. If hands are not carefully and thoroughly washed organisms may be transferred directly to the hand of another or onto objects which will be handled by other people. Equally hazardous would be the transfer of pathogens derived from the bowel to foodstuffs where they may be able to multiply in virtually ideal conditions. Obvious contamination of the fingers is not necessary for this sequence of events to occur. Modern 'absorbent' toilet papers may permit bacteria-bearing moisture to reach the fingers.

After frank diarrhoea, the act of flushing a water closet can generate an aerosol, contaminating the air of the room with infected droplets. Surfaces in a lavatory, such as the toilet seat or the handle of the flushing mechanism, taps, or shelves, may be infected by the 'fall-out', and subsequent users are put at risk of infection by touching infected surfaces or by inhalation or ingestion of droplets. Clearly it is wise for everyone to wash hands after every visit to the toilet — it is but a short journey for the organisms from fingers to mouth.

Improper disposal of faecal matter poses obvious risks. Habitual defaecation on the ground, as occurs in rural areas of developing countries (and to some extent in developed countries where sanitary provision is absent) leaves material exposed to the attentions of other creatures, of which flies are the most dangerous. Badly maintained disposal units such as overflowing or leaking cess pools or septic tanks can lead to contamination of surface waters. Inadequate design of appliances attached to the water main may lead to risks of back siphoning of contaminated water into the mains supply and there have been instances of erroneous connections of waste water pipes to the fresh water supply, leading to serious outbreaks of gastrointenstinal infections. In some countries the use of human faecal material ('night soil') to fertilize crops has been accompanied by the dissemination of parasitic disease.

Contamination of food

Infection may enter food from droplets, from the fingers of an unhygienic cook, it may be carried to the food by flies or other creatures, it may be derived from utensils which have been infected, or it may be present in the food, derived from the carcase of an animal. The infection most commonly transmitted through food is salmonellosis. Salmonella infections of the gut are commonplace in cattle and poultry, and many of these creatures are symptomless carriers. When the animal is slaughtered, some salmonellae may find their way to the carcase meat. Provided the meat is kept refrigerated there is little growth of the bacilli, and once the meat is cooked, it is sterilized. However raw meat may contaminate kitchen equipment — for instance knives which are later used to slice cold cooked meat — and inadequate cooking may permit some infection to remain deep within a joint of meat. Even so, provided the meat is stored at a suitable temperature until eaten, there will be little replication of the few salmonellae present, and those present will be insufficient to cause an infection. If the meat is not kept cool and the bacteria are permitted to multiply, an infectious dose of organisms will accumulate within an hour or two. Environmental conditions are thus a major factor in facilitating the transmission of infection through food and outbreaks of bacterial food poisoning can usually be traced back to a failure of good practice at some point of the food preparation and storage process.

Mechanical transfer by insects and animals

Insects may pick up and carry microorganisms by just walking on infected materials. The main risk of infection is to exposed food. Flies are clearly particularly dangerous because they feed on decaying and faceal matter and can fly directly from such materials to food. Cockroaches may also carry dirt and infection into food. Larger creatures such as mice or rats pose a risk not only because of the microorganisms which can be transferred on feet or fur, but because they themselves may be infected, for instance with salmonellae, and are likely to contaminate foodstuffs with their excretions.

Insect bites

Blood sucking insects are important vectors of several human diseases — mosquitos in the transmission of malaria and filariasis, the tse tse fly in trypanosomiasis, rat fleas in plague, and ticks and mites in typhus.

In all these cases transmission occurs because the insect feeds by taking blood from an infected person or animal, and then feeds on another, injecting some infected material in the process. Because of the influence of environmental factors such as climate and living conditions, the conditions referred to above occur and are transmitted mainly in tropical or subtropical countries, however, there has been some suspicion that bed bugs may transmit serum hepatitis (hepatitis B) in temperate countries, and typhus and plague could also occur anywhere if the conditions are bad enough.

Surgical or quasi-surgical operations

Blood may be transferred from one person to another during processes such as injections, earpiercing or tattooing if inadequate hygiene is practised. The use of the same syringe, let alone the same needle, to give injections to a series of individuals is to be utterly deprecated, and in these days of pre-sterilized disposable equipment is totally unnecessary. Similarly, needles used for tattooing or for earpiercing should be properly cleaned and sterilized between individuals. Serum hepatitis is commonly transmitted if these precautions are not observed. About one person in every thousand in the United Kingdom is an asymptomatic chronic carrier of the hepatitis B virus, and the only way of recognizing such individuals is by special tests. Drug addicts who administer their own drugs by injection and who often share needles and syringes, inadequately sterilized, are known to have a particularly high incidence of serum hepatitis, and are particularly likely to be carriers.

3.3.3 Survival of organisms in the inanimate environment

Unless transference from one living host to the next is immediate, microorganisms have to survive for a period of time in the inanimate environment. Their power to survive, and the presence or absence of factors which will affect that power, are thus of considerable importance in determining whether or not the infection will be successfully transmitted.

Temperature Bacteria and viruses are well able to withstand low temperatures; deep freezing is commonly used for the preservation of cultures. However growth and reproduction can take place only within a relatively restricted range. Beyond this, activity will again cease. Once the temperature rises above 60°C some mortality will occur, and increasing temperature is associated with an increasing mortality rate. Time and temperature act in a complementary way, so that a long exposure to a relatively low temperature will have the same effect as a short exposure to a high temperature. For example, in the pasteurization of milk it is permissible to heat the milk to 63–65.6°C (145–150°F) for 30 minutes, or 72°C (161°F) for 15 seconds, in each case followed by immediate cooling to below 10°C (50°F).

Moist heat has greater penetrating power than dry heat, so is more efficient as a destructive agent. There is considerable variation between species in sensitivity to high temperatures. Some species have the capacity to produce heat resistant spores which will resist a temperature of 100°C for up to 20 minutes. Sterilization implies the complete destruction of all organisms, including heat resistant spores. This requires moist heat at a temperature of up to 120°C if it is to be achieved in a reasonably short period of time, as can be done with an autoclave. Saturated steam reaches a temperature of 120°C under 103.5 kPa (15 lb per sq in) pressure — this will kill most organisms in a period of 30 minutes.

Radiation   Bacteria, viruses and other disease producing microorganisms are destroyed by ionizing radiation such as gamma rays; pre-packed syringes and instruments may be sterilized by such means. Microorganisms are also susceptible to the non-ionizing ultraviolet radiation present in sunlight. The bactericidal wavelengths of ultraviolet are at the shorter, less penetrating end of the ultraviolet spectrum i.e. at wavelengths of 210 to 296 nm, and are reduced in intensity wherever the atmosphere is misty or cloudy. Hence a polluted atmosphere will reduce the bactericidal effect of sunlight. Haemolytic streptococci can be readily demonstrated in dust in the darker areas of a hospital ward when they cannot be found in those places exposed to direct or even diffuse sunlight.

Moisture   Dessication prevents the growth of bacteria and fungi, and is an effective way of preventing food spoilage or the growth of food-poisoning bacteria in food. The organisms are not killed however and are able to resume growth and multiplication when conditions become more favourable.

Chemicals   Detergents such as soap, or certain synthetic detergents (quaternary ammonium compounds) are bactericidal. Most organisms are killed fairly quickly by soap, some within seconds, most within minutes. An effective first aid measure when dealing with a bite from a potentially rabid animal is to wash the wound thoroughly with soapy water. Not all organisms are killed by synthetic detergents, however, and some may actively grow in them. Alcohol at a concentration of 70% is bactericidal, and halogens such as chlorine and iodine will kill organisms but are readily inactivated if organic material, especially protein, is present. Chlorine is extensively used to sterilize water.

Some chemicals have been deliberately developed as disinfectants. Phenols and cresols, derived from coal tar, are useful bactericidal agents provided that they are used at the correct dilutions. The death rate of organisms tends to be high when their numbers are high, but falls geometrically as the numbers fall. If V is the rate of destruction of organisms, and C represents their concentration, then $V = kC$. The constant k is given by the formula

$$k = \frac{1}{t} \log \frac{B}{b}$$

where B represents the initial number of living organisms and b is the number remaining alive after time t (Topley and Wilson, 1975). The graph of mortality rate against time thus takes a negative exponential form, and, in theory, it is never possible to kill every organism present. Hence disinfectants cannot be used for purposes of sterilization.

In everyday life several factors go a long way towards restricting the survival of pathogenic organisms in significant numbers in the environment, and so substantially interfere with the further transmission of communicable disease — cleanliness, preventing the accumulation of dirt which may harbour microorganisms; ventilation, preventing the accumulation of droplets and droplet nuclei; sunlight, allowing ultraviolet radiation to do its work; personal cleanliness, using bactericidal soap or other detergents to reduce the load of bacteria on the skin; keeping food covered and cool to prevent contamination and bacterial growth; and the appropriate use of efficient disinfecting agents when necessary. In those countries where insect transmission is a significant problem, efforts to reduce the breeding potential of insects, and methods of protection against insect bites are of great importance. Control of the intermediate agents in the transmission of parasitic disease to man also makes a significant contribution to disease control. This is the case, for instance, with schistosomiasis, where control of the aquatic snails, the intermediate hosts of the infecting parasite, effectively breaks the chain of transmission to man.

3.3.4 Portal of entry

An organism must enter the body through the appropriate route if it is to have an optimum chance of establishing itself; it should enter the body at such a point that it will arrive with some ease and certainty at its natural habitat. Thus it suffices for staphylococci to reach the surface of the skin, but organisms causing respiratory disease have to be inhaled, and those causing gastrointestinal disease have to be swallowed. The ancient practice of *variolation* (the forerunner of vaccination as protection against smallpox) in which protection was obtained by inoculation of the arm with the pus from another person's smallpox vesicle depended upon the fact that the virus really needed to enter the nasopharynx in order to establish itself as a generalized infection. Infection by a less appropriate route usually resulted in a localized skin infection, and no more.

3.3.5 Factors affecting the outcome of infection

Even if an infecting organism is successfully transmitted to a new host, infection and disease do not necessarily follow. The invading organism has to run the gauntlet of a series of defences if it is to establish itself. There are a number of influences which will affect the outcome, including the infecting dose of organisms, its virulence, and the state of the body's defences.

Infecting dose

The number of organisms comprising the infecting 'dose' is critical — one or two bacilli will fail to establish themselves unless exceptionally virulent, or the victim exceptionally weak. The size of the infecting dose is only one variable in this very complex equation, but, in general terms, some organisms appear to require much larger infecting doses than others. To acquire salmonellosis for instance, it is usually necessary to consume food in which organisms have had a chance to multiply — a culture of the salmonella in fact. This explains why these infections are usually transmitted through food and are not easily acquired simply by personal contact. Where person to person transmission of salmonellae does occur it tends to be in circumstances where there is gross faecal pollution (e.g. incontinence) associated with inadequate general hygiene, or alternatively, where the victim is already debilitated, as in hospital wards. Other diseases require smaller infecting doses to establish themselves; for example dysentery due to *Shigella sonnei* is very readily transmitted and, although it too can be transmitted through infected food, it is much more commonly acquired through contact with an infected environment.

Virulence of the organism

The harm caused by a pathogenic organism growing in the body results from the release of toxic substances. Exotoxins are produced by growing organisms; endo-toxins are only released at their death and dissolution. Some microorganisms pro-duce quite potent exotoxins during their growth which have damaging effects on specific body tissues and may impair the defence mechanisms of the body. Strains which are less efficient toxin producers or grow less rapidly will be correspondingly less efficient invaders and will produce less severe symptoms. The dangerous effects of infection by diphtheria (caused by *Corynebacterium diphtheriae*) are due to its exotoxin. Non-toxigenic strains of this organism circulate in the population with-out causing diphtheria, and are occasionally discovered unexpectedly in throat swabs. The more virulent strains of the streptococcus which caused severe out-breaks of a dangerous variant of scarlet fever a hundred years ago have disappeared; as a result the disease is now much less serious.

State of the body's defences

The defences of the body against infection are arranged in three basic levels: mechanical/chemical; cellular; and humoral.

The first line defences, comprising mechanical or chemical barriers to the entry of microorganisms, are always immediately available. The skin itself is relatively impermeable and organisms cannot pass beyond its surface or the depressions formed by hair follicles unless it is cut or perforated in some way, or unless the in-vaders themselves have some means of boring into it, as does the mite *Sarcoptes scabiei*, or, possibly, certain spirochaetes. Mucous membranes are thinner and have living cells on their surfaces, so are much more prone to attack, especially by viruses which need to enter living cells. However, mucous membranes are usually protected by chemical barriers or layers of mucus which entrap and transport away invading organisms. Often the pH is at a level unsuited to the survival of microorganisms; an obvious example is the acidity of the stomach. The cornea and conjunctiva of the eye are constantly bathed by lachrymal fluid which has mild bactericidal properties, the mucous membrances of the respiratory tract are similarly coated with mucus which is constantly swept away by the action of the cilia lining the bronchi.

If invaders penetrate the first line defences they are attacked within minutes by the second line, cellular, defences of the body. Local cellular damage, perhaps caused by the initial activities of the organisms, or by the trauma which permitted their entry, causes the release of chemical substances which attract local cellular aggregations to surround and wall in the infection. This reaction is typified by the so-called histamine response, visually demonstrated by the simple experiment of drawing a blunt edge, such as the end of a ruler, firmly along the skin of the inner forearm. An instantaneous blanching of the skin caused by preliminary reflex con-striction of the capillaries is followed within seconds by a reddening of the area as the capillaries dilate widely. Plasma leaks out through the capillary walls, increasing the fluid content of the tissues so that a slight swelling develops under the red flare, and as the accumulating fluid masks the dilated capillaries, a white elevated line develops along the centre of the flare. A typical 'wheal' is now present. Micro-scopic examination of the affected region reveals a rapid congregation of leucocytes (white cells). Drifting along in the blood stream in the capillaries they adhere to the wall and then escape through gaps between the wall cells into the increasing pool of tissue fluid. These escaping cells consist of monocytes, which have an immuno-logical function concerned with the humoral defence mechanisms to be mentioned next, and polymorphonuclear leucocytes, which have a scavenging function, attacking and engulfing the invading microorganisms. The invaders are very rapidly surrounded by a hostile cellular environment and may be effectively walled in and even destroyed. Some local cell destruction occurs, and the liquefaction of necrotic tissue may lead to abscess formation.

Some organisms have developed the ability to break down these local defences and may produce a spreading infection. Others produce dangerous exotoxins which circulate in the blood stream throughout the body even though the organism itself is localized. In these events, or if the second line defences fail to destroy the infection rapidly, the third line of defences, which depend upon the production of specific antibodies against the invaders, come into play.

Antibodies are produced by monocytes such as lymphocytes and other cells of the reticulo-endothelial system. Their development depends upon cellular recognition of the protein of the invader as 'foreign'. It takes several days to begin to produce antibodies effectively *ab initio*, and it may be two or three weeks before concentrations appear in the blood which are adequate enough to finally overcome the infection. However, once the technique of producing the specific antibodies required has been learnt, they can be recalled very rapidly even months or years later (*anamnestic response*). Thus some diseases can only successfully infect an individual once, after which a permanent immunity is achieved. Efficient antibody production is a vital part of the body's defence against infection, as may be seen when the ability to produce them is lost or impaired. Patients undergoing transplant surgery, where antibodies against the foreign proteins of implanted organs may develop and destroy them, are given treatment designed to suppress their immunological function, but then have to be cared for in a virtually sterile environment to protect against infection. To a lesser degree, any influences which impair antibody synthesis will undermine resistance to infection. The ability to produce antibodies is dependent upon good general health which, in its turn, is dependent upon the environment in which an individual lives. A particularly important factor is nutrition, especially an adequate intake of protein and vitamins.

3.4 Environment and the risk of infection

The presence or absence of a pathogenic microorganism is, to a large extent, determined by the opportunities which it has to flourish, and the presence and competition of other microorganisms. The presence of dirt and organic detritus in moist conditions provides a potential breeding place of continuing infection. This may apply to the condition of a room or the condition of the body. Personal cleanliness is important because it removes layers of dead cornified cells from the skin, particularly from naturally moist areas of the body in which skin flora may flourish. Similarly, regular changing and cleansing of clothing keeps its bacterial content under control.

The over use of antibiotics which suppress normal (commensal) body flora may, by removing competition, enable other organisms which are relatively insensitive to the antibiotics to grow. For instance, the suppression of the normal flora of the bowel sometimes enables the rapid and excessive multiplication of other organisms causing inflammation of the gut wall and diarrhoea.

It is clearly important to reduce the size of reservoirs of infection as much as possible; if a reservoir can be totally eliminated, the infection may be eradicated. This has actually happened with the disease smallpox, for the only reservoir of this infection was active human infection. Surprisingly little public attention was paid to this remarkable achievement, finally confirmed by the World Health Organization in May 1980. One of the most dreaded diseases of mankind once widespread throughout the world, had been wiped off the face of the earth — and most people hardly noticed (see Fig. 3.8).

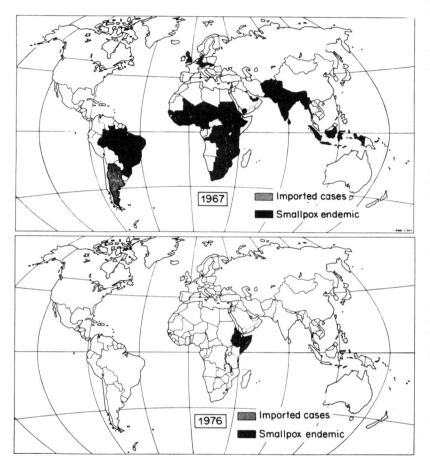

Fig. 3.8   The extent of smallpox in the world in 1967 and 1976. The last recorded case of smallpox in the world (apart from the case in Birmingham which was caused by a laboratory virus) was diagnosed in Somalia in October 1977. (Maps reproduced from the *Weekly Epidemiological Record*, 25 April 1980, No. 17, with the permission of the World Health Organization.)

As far as the multitude of diseases still in existence are concerned, prompt recognition of cases will allow precautions to be taken to prevent further transmission and rapid and effective treatment will remove the risk from that case for good. The recognition of the case can also lead to a search for its source, which, if not already harmless, can be rendered so. In order to facilitate the application of these processes by those responsible, many important communicable diseases are statutorily notifiable to the local authority. There is extensive legislation relating to the powers of local authorities and their officers (Table 3.7). As well as overt cases, it is important to identify short term or long term carriers and to place appropriate constraints on their activities, where necessary, to prevent them from infecting others. Often

Table 3.7 The principal Acts and Regulations related to the control of communicable disease.

Public Health Act 1936 (Part V)
Food Act 1984
Milk and Dairies (General) Regulations 1959
Public Health Act 1961
Public Health (Leprosy) Regulations 1966
Health Services and Public Health Act 1968
Public Health (Infectious Diseases) Regulations 1968 and 1985
The Imported Food Regulations 1968, together with Amendment regulations 1973
The Public Health (Ships) Regulations 1970, together with Amendment regulations in 1978
The Public Health (Aircraft) Regulations 1970, together with Amendment regulations in 1978
Public Health (Food Hygiene) Regulations 1970
Public Health (Infectious Diseases) (Amendment) Regulations 1974
Rabies Act 1974
Public Health (Control of Disease) Act 1984

these constraints do not need to be severe. It is usually sufficient to ensure that carriers are fully informed and understand the appropriate precautions that they should take. Carriers of the organism responsible for typhoid fever (*Salmonellae typhi*), for instance, should not work in the food preparation trade or in the water supply industry in jobs which might bring them into contact with mains water. Such persons should, preferably, live in houses with modern sanitation connected to the mains sewerage system. They should refrain from handling food intended for consumption by others; they should practice careful toilet hygiene; and members of their household should be protected with typhoid vaccine. Apart from these precautions, typhoid carriers should lead normal lives; it is inappropriate to exclude them from work or school, since, provided the simple rules given above are obeyed, they will pose no risk to the public at large.

Animal reservoirs of infection can be reduced by ensuring that sick animals are identified and either treated or slaughtered. Cooperation between the medical and veterinary professions in cross-notifying infections of interest to both is becoming more effectively organized through links between Divisional Veterinary Officers, Environmental Health Officers, and Medical Officers for Environmental Health working for local authorities. Animal carriers of infection can be reduced by removing infected animals from herds and mounting eradication campaigns similar to those for the eradication of tuberculosis and brucellosis in cattle. Domestic animals should be kept in clean conditions and regularly treated to eliminate parasites such as fleas and worm infestations. It is in the owner's interest, as well as that of the animal, to maintain it in a healthy and disease free condition.

Risks of transmission of infection are enhanced by proximity to an infectious case. Hence, in the case of dangerous and highly infectious diseases, actual isolation or quarantine of the case is necessary, and those who must come into proximity to the case should wear protective clothing. Such extreme measures are usually undertaken only in respect of diseases such as the viral haemorrhagic fevers and possibly the enteric fevers. Droplet infection can be minimized by avoiding very close proximity to cases as far as possible, avoiding overcrowding of rooms, and ensuring good ventilation so that effective dilution and dispersal of droplets and droplet nuclei to the open air can occur. Good hygiene on the part of those infected, by suppressing the spray from coughs and sneezes by effective use of handkerchiefs is also most important. The potential danger of infectious organisms lurking in dust can be reduced by adequate dust control measures, especially the regular use of vacuum cleaners, and by having light sunny rooms where ultraviolet light can be effective. Careful maintenance and regular cleaning of humidifiers will help to reduce the dangers of humidifer fever or Legionnaires disease.

The spread of gastrointenstinal infections is facilitated by inefficient sanitation and bad personal toilet hygiene. Wash hand basins and soap and towels should be easily available for use after visiting the toilet; for public places, individual paper towels or 'dispensed' continuous linen towels should be available. Roller towels should never be used. Alternatively, hot air dryers may be provided. Water closets connected to a main sewerage system should be provided wherever possible. Septic tanks or cess pools must be properly maintained, and proper arrangements should be made for the regular emptying of chemical closets where these are in use. It should never be necessary to use earth closets, which are potentially dangerous through the encouragement and potential infection of flies. Good food hygiene is also important, to prevent the spread of infection through food. Persons suffering from bowel infections, even if only carriers, should never prepare food intended for consumption for others. All prepared food should be kept covered until consumed, and food containing protein should be stored at temperatures below $4°C$ or above $60°C$ and should, whenever possible, be consumed as soon as it has been cooked. Cooking techniques must also be adequate, to ensure full heat penetration and hence sterilization of the food. This especially applies to meat and poultry and, in particular, to deep frozen products, which must be completely thawed before cooking commences. Every Christmas there are a number of outbreaks of salmonella infection associated with the consumption of poultry which has not adequately thawed before being placed in the oven.

Susceptibility to infection is increased if nutrition is generally poor and if there is undue exposure to fatigue or extreme temperatures, especially cold. That the relatively undernourished succumb more readily to infectious diseases and their complications is amply demonstrated in many developing countries. In some African states, for instance, measles is a much more lethal disease than it is in the United Kingdom. Protein malnutrition particularly undermines the ability to formulate an adequate antibody response. A good balanced diet, containing sufficient protein and vitamins, together with trace elements, will ensure that ability to fight off invading organisms is at its optimum.

Some members of a population may lack natural immunity to a disease because they have never been in contact with it. Experimental studies using animal colonies have demonstrated how repetitive epidemic waves may occur in populations where there is a steady accumulation of non-immune susceptibles until a 'flash-point' is reached. A large epidemic follows, leaving a high proportion of the surviving population immune. The process then repeats itself as new generations of non-immunes are added. In human populations this phenomenon has been seen in the biennial peaks of measles epidemics and the four yearly cycles of whooping cough outbreaks. However, immunity may be stimulated arti-ficially by the use of suitable vaccines. If a large proportion of the population can be kept immune the probability of an infectious person meeting a sus-ceptible person is reduced. With highly infectious diseases such as measles and whooping cough it is necessary to attain a state where some 90% of the population is immune if transmission is to be effectively interrupted.

3.4.1   The effects of the social environment

Human behaviour affects the occurrence of communicable disease by enhanc-ing opportunities for transmission to occur. Improvements in social con-ditions, especially the improvement of living conditions, so that it is possible to live more hygienically, and nutrition, so that resistance to infection is optimum, play their part. But they cannot be effective unless, through the effects of education, those at risk are able to take full advantage of the improved conditions, and, further, are willing to do so. Inadequate diet, in-sufficient rest, the abuse of alcohol or drugs will continue to undermine bodily health and enhance the risks of infection.

Examples of the effects of social change on the occurrence of communic-able diseases are not hard to find. Tuberculosis has always been strongly associated with adverse social conditions, and pockets of infection still persist in socially disadvantaged groups such as alcoholics and vagrants, although it has shown a sharp decline in the population in general. Mortality from tuber-culosis fell sharply once the anti-tuberculosis drugs were discovered, but the morbidity caused by the disease, as demonstrated by notification rates, has responded much less dramatically to the introduction of effective drugs. Indeed, as Fig. 3.9 shows, the fall in incidence of pulmonary tuberculosis which started during the nineteenth century, has shown surprisingly little fluctuation in response to the introduction of various medical measures in-troduced with the objective of controlling it during this century, and indeed it appears to have continued inexorably almost in spite of them. This disease, which was a scourge in the past, will soon be relatively rare in the United Kingdom, although it will persist elsewhere in the world where social con-ditions are less conducive to its disappearance and doubtless will continue to occur in socially disadvantaged groups in this country.

Sexual promiscuity and prostitution maintain the transmission of venereal disease (VD). With the advent of penicillin the medical profession was able to glimpse the possibility of conquering gonorrhoea. After the second world war the disease declined considerably in incidence and there was much opti-mism that it might be brought under control. However, in company with several other indices of the effects of social change, this infection has in-creased considerably in incidence since the mid 1950s until it is now again very common. The situation is complicated by the emergence of penicillin resistant strains of the gonococcus. This re-emergence of an infection which is entirely dependent upon human behaviour for its transmission, has been accompanied by such changes as increased frankness about sexual matters, with regular portrayal in some detail of sexual encounters in films, television

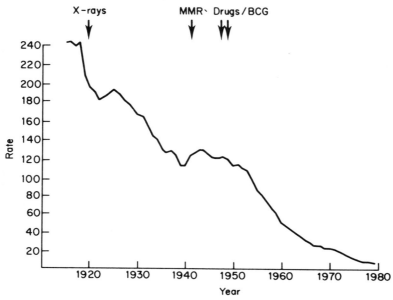

Fig. 3.9   Tuberculosis in England and Wales. Notification rates per 100 000. (Data from OPCS.)

and plays, an increased proportion of women going out to work leading to greater mixing of the sexes, and the introduction of oral contraception, which removes the need for barrier methods which to some extent hinder the transmission of infection. The advent of antibiotics — the means of an easy and rapid cure for anyone unlucky enough to become infected — may itself have contributed to a 'laissez faire' attitude towards the risk of VD in some persons.

4
Cancer

4.1   Aspects of epidemiology

Cancer is an uncontrolled growth of a group of cells in the body. The cells lose their functional differentiation and begin to reproduce themselves indiscriminately, overgrowing their natural boundaries, distorting their surroundings, and destroying the normally ordered structure of the tissues in which they are growing. Secondary growths occur elsewhere in the body, disseminated from the primary growth by cells which separate off and are swept away to new locations by the blood stream or in the flow of lymphatic fluid through lymph channels and lymph nodes. Sooner or later the growing masses of cells interfere with the function of a vital organ of the body, or the growth itself outgrows its own blood supply and becomes necrotic. The breakdown of the tissues may then lead to bleeding and secondary infection. Eventually the life of the victim is destroyed by organ failure, or infection, or by massive haemorrhage. Sometimes the sheer inanition caused by the growth leads to exhaustion and death.

Cancer is one of the most important causes of modern mortality, especially in the developed countries, where the risk of death from communicable disease has been largely eliminated. Although it is popularly associated with old age — and indeed the risk of developing cancer increases steadily with age — it can occur at all ages and is, for instance, second only to accidents as a cause of death in children. Cancer is primarily classified according to the system of the body which is affected, the particular organ within that system and the kind of tissue from which the growth is derived. Figure 4.1 illustrates the death rates from the commoner forms of cancer in England and Wales in such a way that the occurrence of each type may be seen in perspective and in relation to that of the others. The diagram also illustrates the differential incidence in the sexes. Certain general characteristics are apparent. In most bodily systems the death rates of males exceed those of females. This relationship is reversed only in the case of cancers affecting the reproductive system and breast. The very great importance of cancer of the lung in men is obvious.

Although cancer is by no means confined to older age groups and certain kinds are a major cause of death in children, the incidence of the disease rises with age in both sexes (Fig. 4.2). Experimental studies have shown that exposure to carcinogenic agents needs to continue for a period of time, and that tissues may go through recognizable pre-cancerous changes before the definitive lesion appears, so that cancer has a recognizable induction period. In some instances, careful observations of the occurrence of cancer in humans after exposure to identified environmental factors have shown that the induction period may extend into many years. This

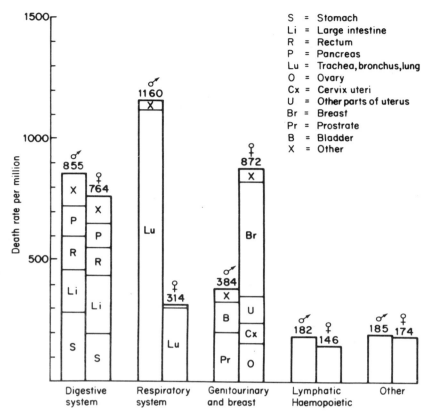

Fig. 4.1   Death rates per million from cancer in England and Wales, 1978. (Data from OPCS.)

may be one explanation for the more common occurrence of the condition in the later years of life.

The science of epidemiology looks for significant 'associations' between the occurrence of specific factors, usually environmental, and the occurrence of a given disease. If factor and disease are found to be associated more frequently than would be expected on a purely random or chance basis, a 'significant' association is said to exist. An association may be deemed to be direct or indirect in nature; if it is direct, it may or may not be causal. The mere finding of a significant association is not, in rigorously scientific terms, proof of a causal association, although the finding is likely to stimulate researchers into seeking to investigate its nature in cosiderable depth.

4.1.1   Geographical distribution of cancer

The incidence of cancer varies from place to place. Differences in occurrence may be observed on an international scale, within individual countries, where certain parts may show varying rates of occurrence, or between particular types of locality, such as the variations which are observed between urban and rural populations. There are, however, certain problems about ascertaining the true incidence of cancer. The most easily obtainable data relates to mortality. Clearly the accuracy

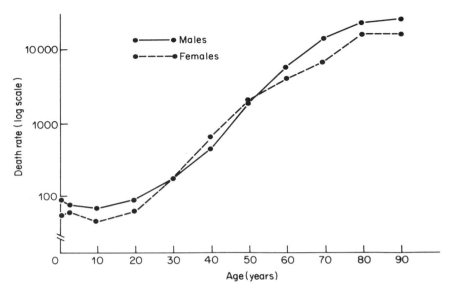

Fig. 4.2 Death rates per million from all forms of cancer; by age and sex, England and Wales, 1978. (Data from OPCS.)

of mortality as a proxy indicator of the incidence of cancer depends upon the case fatality rate, which itself may be partly dependent upon the efficiency with which early diagnosis is achieved and the effectiveness of the treatment employed. International comparisons may be influenced by variations in the provision of medical services. Such sources of error are less important when comparing incidence within different parts of the same country. Morbidity statistics are available in some countries, for example, in the United Kingdom, detailed information can be extracted from Hospital Activity Analysis (HAA) files, and the OPCS publishes occasional supplements on cancer.

Provided adequate allowances are made for such sources of error, geographical variations in incidence may be examined to see whether they are statistically significant; if they are, they require explanation. Variations of a geographical nature affecting large areas or whole countries may arise from genetic variation between the peoples living in different parts of the world, or they may reflect the differential effects of environmental factors. These two potential groups of causes – genetic and environmental – can be separated by observing the effects of migration. Where a true geographical (environmental) association exists the high incidence rates occur in all the inhabitants of the region, whatever their racial or ethnic origin; similar high frequencies are not observed in similar groups outside the region. Healthy persons coming to reside in the region come to experience a similar incidence of the condition whereas those who leave it cease to suffer the relatively high incidence noted there.

Such relationships have been found to occur with certain kinds of cancer; they are highly suggestive of environmental influences, physical or social, but there are considerable difficulties in discovering just what these are. Most of the associations remain unexplained, although various hypotheses have been advanced. Zones of high incidence of cancer of the oesophagus can be identified. It is relatively common, for instance, amongst the Africans of South Africa. Yet, although the death rate amongst these people is one per thousand per annum, it is as low as 25 per million in other parts of the same continent. Cancer of the oesophagus also occurs very commonly in Iran. On the whole, rates on the continent of Europe are relatively low, although the death rate in France is slightly elevated.

Cancer of the stomach shows quite remarkable geographical variations in incidence; in global terms, the death rate from this cause is high in the Far East, especially in Japan, and tends to decline as one moves away on the other side of the globe, being lowest in the U.S.A. (Fig. 4.3). Within the United Kingdom there are

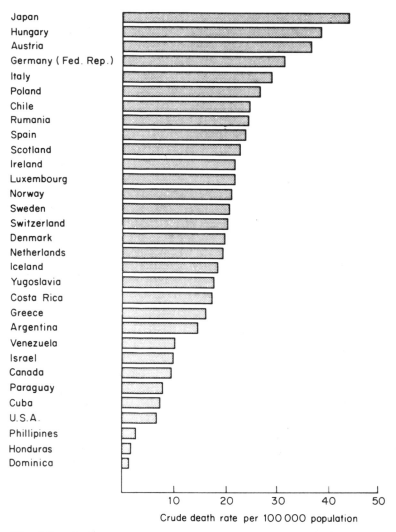

Fig. 4.3   Global mortality from stomach cancer. (Data from *World Health Organization Statistics Annual* (1980). World Health Organization.)

areas of particularly high incidence, for instance in North West Wales. Cancer of the colon tends to show an inverse distribution to that of stomach cancer.

Primary liver cancer is not amongst the more common cancers in the U.K., although the liver is a favourite site for the occurrence of secondary cancer. However, there are foci of primary liver cancer incidence in Africa, traced to the influence of a known carcinogen, aflatoxin, which occurs in mouldy ground nuts. There is also an increased risk of developing primary liver cancer after an attack of serum hepatitis, especially if a chronic infection supervenes. Since there is a relatively high incidence of serum hepatitis in Africa, this also may be making a contribution.

Cancer of the breast tends to be commoner in Western countries. It shows a relatively high incidence in parts of North America. A decreasing incidence northwards through the British Isles and Scandinavia has also been reported. Britain, and particularly Scotland, has the unenviable distinction of having one of the highest rates of lung cancer in the world. High rates are also found in the U.S.A., Northern Europe, and Australasia.

4.1.2   Cancer and occupation

Many instances of the association of some kinds of cancer with specific occupations have been documented. The first occupational cancer to be so recognized was cancer of the scrotum, described by Percival Pott in 1775, which occurred in chimney sweeps due to exposure to soot. Since then, numerous associations have been recognized, and indeed are still coming to light (Table 4.1). The discovery of these associations has led to the identification of materials which are capable of stimulating the appearance of cancer of specific sites if exposure is frequent and prolonged enough. The induction period often extends to many years; for instance, mesothelioma of the pleura (a form of cancer affecting the lung) has occurred up to forty years after exposure to crocidolite asbestos.

4.1.3   Social class distribution of cancer

The linkage of variations in incidence with occupational risks will affect the social class distribution of cancer, but differential social class distributions may also indicate the effects of varying physical environments or of socially determined behavioural factors as discussed in Chapter 2. This latter effect is well illustrated in the linkage of cigarette smoking and lung cancer (see pp. 59—60).

4.1.4   Distribution in time

Changes in the incidence of a cancer as time progresses may be seen to accompany or follow upon a change in exposure to a possible environmental factor. Clearly such a finding must be treated with circumspection; the mere fact that two events are synchronous or sequential does not necessarily mean that they are causally related. Certain criteria must be fulfilled before a causal relationship may be reasonably suspected; the time sequence and any hypothetical relationship must be compatible with existing knowledge, and with other observations.

4.2   Lung cancer

Figure 4.1 clearly illustrates the importance of lung cancer as the major single contributor to cancer mortality in the United Kingdom. Some 6% of all deaths in England and Wales are currently due to this condition (9% of male deaths).

Table 4.1   Occupational cancer.

Cancer sites	Related occupations	Carcinogenic agents
Scrotum	Chimney sweeps (historical)	Coal tar derivatives,
	Lathe and machine tool workers	especially 3.4 benzyprene
	Tar and pitch workers	Mineral oils
	Cotton mule spinners	
Skin	Lathe and machine tool operators	Aromatic hydrocarbons
	Tar and pitch workers	
	Outdoor workers	Ultraviolet radiation
Lungs	Gas house workers	Aromatic hydrocarbons
	Foundry workers	
	Chemical workers	Chloromethyl methyl ether
		Arsenic
	Asbestos workers	Asbestos, especially
		crocidolite
	Nickle and chromium workers	Nickle, chromium fumes
	Uranium miners	Radon
	Haematite miners	Iron oxide
Nasal sinuses	Hardwood workers	Hardwood dust
	Leather workers	Leather dust
	Chromium and nickle refiners	Chromium and nickle fumes
Bladder	Tar and pitch workers	Aromatic hydrocarbons
	Gas house workers	
	Dye manufacturers	Coal tar derivatives
	Rubber workers	
	Leather and shoe workers	
Liver	Workers in the plastics industry	Vinyl chloride
	Tanners	Arsenic
	Smelters	

Mortality from lung cancer, as measured by SMRs, is greater in urban than in rural areas. The SMRs are particularly raised in the industrial towns of South Wales, the Midlands, and the North West. As is usually the case with environmental matters, it seems likely that a number of factors act synergistically in bringing about this raised urban mortality. Thus the general pollution of the atmosphere by the products of combustion of bituminous coal and other fuels, combined with the escape of industrial fumes, is accompanied by an increased likelihood of exposure to occupations which are known to carry an increased risk of lung cancer. Pollution of the atmosphere, especially by the smoke generated by the inefficient combustion of coal, is accompanied by the presence of known carcinogens such as 3,4 benzpyrene in the atmosphere. Much has been achieved through the application of the Clean Air Acts to reduce the amount of atmospheric pollution, but the existence of large conurbations side by side with industries such as smelting works and foundries inevitably leads to heavier pollution of the atmosphere than would be found in the countryside or on the moors.

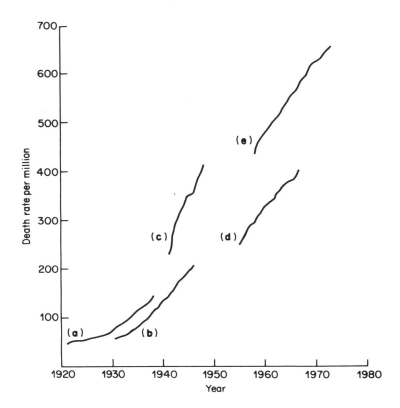

Fig. 4.4 The death rate from cancer of the lung has increased fifteen fold over the last fifty years. The graph illustrates the climb in the death rate which started in the mid-twenties. The discontinuity of the graph is due to the variety of definitions which have been used in the ICCD over the years: (a) cancer of respiratory organs; (b) cancer of lung and pleura; (c) cancer of trachea, bronchus and lung; (d) cancer of bronchus and trachea, and of lung specified as primary; (e) cancer of trachea, bronchus and lung. (Data from various Registrar Generals and OPCS tabulations.)

The way in which the occurrence of lung cancer has changed during the 20th century is quite remarkable, and its rise in incidence during the past sixty years may be viewed as having reached epidemic proportions. Figure 4.4 shows how the death rate has risen from about 40 per million in the 1920s to nearly 700 per million at the present time. The rise has occurred differentially in the sexes, starting first in men around 1926, but not appearing to a significant extent in women until the 1950s. It is almost certainly of considerable significance that these changes in the occurrence of lung cancer followed upon similar changes in the distribution of cigarette smoking between the sexes (see Fig. 8.4). The burning of wood, and later of coal, has gone on for centuries, and men and women have been equally affected by it. Towns and cities came into existence at the time of the industrial revolution, as did many of the occupations which are recognized as associated with an increased incidence of lung cancer. None of these factors has changed dramatically during this century, but the consumption of cigarettes has. The polluting effect of cigarettes is considered in more detail in Chapter 8; suffice it to note here that men began to smoke cigarettes in significant quantities around the turn of the century, whereas women did not take up the habit in any numbers until just before and during the second world war. This time difference can be seen to be related to the differential timing in the onset of the lung cancer epidemic in men and women. In each case there is an interval of about 30 years, which may be related to the induction period which is a feature of the development of many cancers. These time relationships are highly suggestive of a cause and effect relationship.

The rise in cancer in women was predictable. In 1960, it was possible to write 'It is now some forty years since women began to smoke, but in the early 1920s only very few did so, and they did not begin to smoke in appreciable numbers until the mid and late 1930s . . . . On this basis one would expect to see the early signs of an increase in the incidence of lung cancer (in women) about now, and one would expect the incidence in women to increase until it reached a maximum during the 1970s, assuming that female smoking habits continue in their present trends. There are signs that this prophecy is beginning to be fulfilled.' (A.J. Rowland, DPH dissertation, unpublished). Indeed the prophecy has been fulfilled. During the 1970s the incidence of female lung cancer has made the major contribution to the continuing rise in overall cancer mortality.

As will be seen from Table 4.1, certain occupations are known to be associated with an increased risk of developing lung cancer. Some are associated with exposure to fumes from the combustion of coal in coke ovens, or from the smelting of metals, especially nickle and chromium. The effects of irradiation by radon are believed to be the important factor in uranium mining. Exposure to asbestos is associated with an increased risk of lung cancer — a risk which is potentiated if there is concomitant exposure to cigarette smoke. Also associated with exposure to asbestos is mesothelioma, affecting the pleural membrane surrounding the lung. Although much less common than cancer affecting the bronchi of the lungs it appears to be becoming more common. Table 4.2 shows the number of deaths each year from cancer affecting the pleura. These are not specifically defined as mesothelioma but the steady increase is of interest in view of the increase in the incidence of mesothelioma which has been noted in several studies. Wagner, Slegg and Marchand (1960)

Table 4.2   Number of deaths from neoplasms of the pleura in England and Wales for the years 1968 to 1978. (Data from OPCS.)

Year	Males	Females
1968	96	39
1969	92	36
1970	110	46
1971	89	39
1972	107	36
1973	127	36
1974	115	50
1975	159	41
1976	166	43
1977	178	51
1978	199	41

described the occurrence of mesothelioma of the pleura in patients exposed to croc-idolite asbestos in association with mining in the Cape Province, South Africa. This well documented study indicates a history of contact with asbestos in nearly all the cases. By the end of June 1960 a total of 47 cases of mesothelioma had been identi-fied, and in 45 of these a possible association with exposure to crocidolite had been established. According to these workers, the first recorded case of carcinoma of the lungs associated with asbestos was described in 1935, and two cases of diffuse mesothelioma from a chrysotile mine were described by Cartier in 1952.

In a study of 83 Londoners with confirmed mesothelioma, Newhouse and Thompson (1965) found that half of them gave a history of occupational or dom-estic contact with asbestos. Of those with no such history, one third lived within half a mile of an asbestos factory. The interval between first exposure and the development of the terminal illness ranged between 16 and 55 years. Asbestos or asbestos bodies (a local cellular reaction to the presence of asbestos) were seen in the tissues of many of the cases.

Lung cancer has its highest incidence in social classes IV and V (see Table 2.4). This distribution can be attributed to a number of factors. Firstly there are occu-pational risks which would affect specific social groups. Secondly, a large propor-tion of those in social classes IV and V live in urban industrial areas where they are more exposed to atmospheric pollution.

Another undoubtedly important factor is the relatively greater consumption of cigarettes by social classes IV and V. A vast amount of evidence has accumulated linking the consumption of cigarettes with an increased risk of developing lung cancer. Early suspicions that lung cancer might be associated with smoking arose in the 1920s. An early case history study carried out by F.H. Muller in Cologne just before the start of the second world war gave impetus to these suspicions. He com-pared the smoking habits of lung cancer victims with those of patients who needed treatment for chest injuries and found that on average the lung cancer victims tended to be heavier smokers. After the war, in the early fifties, a series of similar studies confirmed that an association appeared to exist. However, epidemiologists are suspicious of case history studies because they have inbuilt risks of bias. A clear need to identify smokers who were apparently well, and to follow them up to observe their subsequent disease experience, that is to carry out prospective studies, emerged.

E.C. Hammond and D.H.Horn, and H.F. Dorn, in the United States of America, and R. Doll and A. Bradford Hill in the United Kingdom, all embarked upon such studies independently, and their reports appeared in the medical press in the mid and late fifties. All the studies showed that cigarette smokers had a greater risk of dying at any age than non-smokers and that, although the increased mortality was due to an increased risk of succumbing to a number of diseases, the risk of develop-ing lung cancer was found to be twenty times that of persons of equivalent age who had never smoked. Numerous studies of the relationship between cigarette smoking and lung cancer have revealed a series of facts about the effects of smoking cigar-ettes, all of which point to them as an important agent in enhancing the risk of lung cancer (Table 4.3).

In the face of all this evidence, few would now doubt that if it were possible for everyone to stop smoking cigarettes tomorrow, in ten years time the incidence of lung cancer would have been reduced ten-fold, or possibly even more.

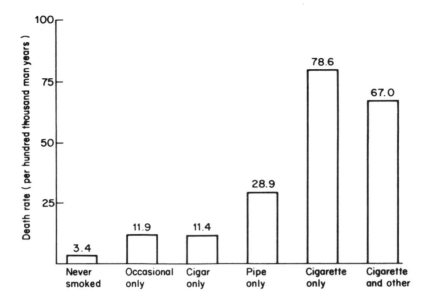

Fig. 4.5   Lung cancer incidence by mode of smoking. Age standardized death rates for well established cases of bronchogenic epithelial carcinoma by type of smoking as established from life history. (From Hammond, E.C. and Horn, D.H. (1958). *Journal of the American Medical Association,* **166,** 1294. ©1958, American Medical Association.)

4.3   Cancer of the cervix

The cervix is the 'neck' of the womb (uterus), which protrudes slightly into the top of the vagina. Cancer develops, in some women, just within the canal joining the exterior opening to the interior of the uterus. The development of a frankly invasive cancer of this site is preceded by changes in the appearance of the cells forming the lining of the canal. The cells may develop all the characteristics of cancerous cells except the over-growth and invasiveness of local tissues. This non-invasive, precancerous, stage is known as 'carcinoma-*in-situ*'. Its existence, and that of less dramatic, but possibly pre-malignant, changes can be discovered by examining a sample of the lining cells, shed naturally from the epithelium of the cervical canal. The sample is obtained by taking a scraping from the entrance to the cervical canal and making a smear of the cells on a glass slide for microscopic examination – the so-called 'cervical smear'.

Studies have shown that not all carcinomas *in situ* progress to frank malignancy, indeed some must regress completely (Table 4.4). Those that do become true cancer may take many years to do so. If a carcinoma *in situ* is discovered it can be destroyed before malignancy can develop. This is a prime example of the patient who is in the third category of the disease spectrum shown in Fig. 1.1 (*q.v.*) and a good opportunity for secondary prevention as described in Chapter 1.

About 2000 women die each year from cancer of the cervix in England and Wales. As Fig. 4.1 demonstrates, this cancer is not one of the most important from a purely numerical point of view, but it is important as an example of a cancer

Table 4.3   Relationship between cigarette smoking and the incidence of lung cancer.

(*i*)   Time relationships, see p. 60.

(*ii*)   Smoking of tobacco as cigarettes is more likely to be followed by lung cancer. The much lower risk experienced by pipe smokers is to some extent offset by their greater propensity to develop lip or tongue cancers (see (*v*)).

(*iii*)   International comparisons have shown that the incidence of lung cancer in a country bears a direct linear relationship to the total amount of tobacco smoked there as cigarettes.

(*iv*)   Both in the U.S.A. and Japan, mortality from lung cancer is lower than would be expected from their levels of cigarette tobacco consumption. R. Doll and A. Bradford Hill have suggested that in the U.S.A. this might be related to the tendency of Americans to smoke less of a cigarette than in some other countries. A comparison showed that in America an average of 40% of the cigarette remained unsmoked; in the U.K. only about 25% was thrown away. The remaining portion of the cigarette acts as a filter, retaining some of the tar — the larger the remaining length of cigarette, the less tar would be absorbed by the smoker.

(*v*)   The tar distillates from tobacco have been shown, in animal experiments, to contain carcinogenic substances. When smoking cigarettes there is a greater chance of the distillates reaching the bronchi because of the temperature of combustion of the tobacco and the steady consumption of the length of the cigarette in which some of the earlier distillate will have condensed. In pipe smokers, much of the tars distil out in the stem and bowl of the pipe. There can be few pipe smokers who have not experienced the unpleasant effects of liquid from the pipe entering the mouth, so allowing potentially carcinogenic substances to come into direct contact with its tissues.

(*vi*)   The risk of developing lung cancer is substantially greater in those cigarette smokers who inhale the smoke.

(*vii*)   The longer a person has smoked, the greater is their risk of developing lung cancer. If a person gives up smoking, the risk of developing lung cancer is reduced and becomes less as the duration of the period of non-smoking increases, until after about ten years, the risk approaches that of a person who has never smoked.

Table 4.4   Rate of reversion of carcinoma *in situ* to cancer of the cervix (based on follow up of 127 subjects). (Adapted from Petersen, O. (1956). *American Journal of Obstetrics and Gynaecology, 72*, 1063—71.)

Follow up period (years)	Number remaining under surveillance	Evidence of regression of histology to normal		Clinical carcinoma of cervix developed	
		No.	%	No.	%
1	127	25	19.7	5	3.9
3	127	30	23.6	14	11.0
5	104	27	16.4	23	22.0
7	64	16	25.0	17	26.6
9	42	10	23.8	14	33.3

which is susceptible, not only to secondary prevention, but also, in theory at least, to primary prevention, for there is much evidence of the influence of environmental factors on its occurrence.

Fabien Gagnon reported in 1949 to a meeting of the Society of Obstetricians and Gynaecologists in Canada that he had carried out a series of careful and systematic searches to determine the incidence of cancer of the cervix in nuns. In his first search he examined the medical records of an annual average of 13 000 nuns, going back over a period of twenty years, and found not a single case. A search of hospital pathology laboratory notes, and of notes held at radium treatment centres, uncovered three microscopically confirmed cases, when he would have expected to find 114. Finally, he looked at the total cancer experience of an annual average of 3280 women, again looking back through 20 years of records, and, although he identified 130 cases of various kinds of cancer in the nuns (including 53 cases of breast cancer) he did not find a single case of cancer of the cervix.

Another group of women who have a remarkably low incidence of cervical cancer are Jewish women, irrespective of which country they inhabit, or to which particular ethnic group they belong. A study carried out in Israel (Hochman, Ratzkowski and Schrieber, 1955) confirmed the results of many previous studies dating back to 1901. The incidence recorded was 2.2 cases per 100 000 Jewish women per annum, which compared with 28 per 100 000 *total population* in Copenhagen, or 39.3 per 100 000 females in Detroit. Haenszel and Hillhouse (1959) reported an incidence of 4.7 per 100 000 Jewish women per annum in New York, compared with an overall rate in the same place of 18.3 per 100 000. In similar studies, Moslem women have also been found to have a relatively low incidence. Although circumcision of their husbands was at one time thought to be a possible common factor in Jewish and Moslem women, subsequent studies on the association of cancer of the cervix with this particular factor in groups where husbands could be either circumcised or not circumcised have failed to confirm its relevance. It would seem that the true factor concerned is most likely to be related to abstinence or restriction of the frequency of sexual intercourse, and restriction of the number of sexual partners which a woman might have. Sexual behaviour in both Jews and Moslems is strictly controlled by their religious laws. They are thus protected from many of the behavioural factors, summarized in Beral (1974) where many supporting references are given, and here in Table 4.5, which have been found to be associated with an enhanced risk of developing cancer of the cervix.

Examination of the relationship between human sexual behaviour and cancer of the cervix leads to the hypothesis that it is associated with the sexual transmission of an infectious agent. A possible candidate has been identified, although there is

Table 4.5   Factors identified as being positively associated with an enhanced risk of developing cancer of the cervix.

Being married	Early age at first intercourse
Broken marriage	Multiple sexual partners
Multiple marriages	Prostitution
Early age at first marriage	Infection with venereal disease
Extramarital sexual activity	Illegitimacy
Premarital sexual activity	Low socioeconomic status
	Urban residence

still considerable controversy about its role. The possibility that the herpes simplex viruses might be implicated was first published by Rawls *et al.* (1968). Some laboratories have reported finding antibody to viral antigens in the serum of cervical cancer patients, but not in the serum of control patients (similar women who were not affected by cancer). Traces of herpes simplex virus nucleic acids have been detected in cancer cells. But these facts do not necessarily mean that the virus causes the cancer. It may be present only as a 'passenger' — perhaps because the cancer cells are particularly prone to infection with this particular group of viruses.

However, if sexually transmitted viruses are the cause of cancer of the cervix, it might be expected that the use of barrier methods of contraception such as the condom or dutch cap would interfere with transmission and reduce the incidence of the disease. But then the converse would be true; decreasing the use of barrier methods would lead to a risk that the incidence of cervical cancer would increase. So would an increase in sexual 'permissiveness'. It may therefore be of some significance that, since the arrival of the 'pill', the incidence of cancer of the cervix in younger women has shown an upward trend, although until comparatively recently there has been an overall tendency for the number of cases to decline from year to year, a decline which began well before the inception of cervical smears.

Cancer of the cervix is undoubtedly a good example of ways in which the occurrence of cancer can be linked with factors in the environment. In this case the factors are social and strongly related to human culture and behaviour. It is possible to identify groups of women who are at greater risk than others — an example of the 'high risk groups' of the disease spectrum (Fig. 1.1). These are the women who should be particularly encouraged to attend regularly for cervical smears. Furthermore, it would perhaps be possible to undertake primary prevention of cancer of the cervix if it were possible to induce changes in the sexual behaviour of the nation, so reducing the 'risk' behaviour.

4.4   Cancer of the stomach

Figure 4.1 demonstrates the relative importance of cancer of the digestive tract as a cause of death from malignant disease, and shows that, of the various forms of digestive tract cancer, cancer of the stomach makes the major contribution. The crude death rate from this condition has fallen steadily in both sexes since the 1940s, suggesting that there has been a true decrease in incidence in the United Kingdom. The social class distribution of stomach cancer mortality indicates an increased risk in the less skilled groups in the community (Fig. 4.6).

The remarkable, and so far unexplained, geographical variation in incidence of stomach cancer, which can be seen both globally and within individual countries, has already been mentioned. Doll (1967) has described a gradient in mortality, with death rates tending to decrease as one progresses westwards from Japan across the Asian and European continents, or eastwards across the Pacific, to the lowest rates, which occur in the U.S.A. Migration studies have tended to discount genetic factors in the relatively high Japanese incidence, for Japanese migrants to the U.S.A. show reduced rates, and the reductions bear a positive relationship to the duration of residence in the U.S.A. For instance, American studies published in 1968 demonstrated that U.S. born citizens with Japanese ancestry suffered only a third of the stomach cancer mortality of Japanese living in Japan, and that those Japanese residing in the U.S.A. who had been born in Japan had just over half the

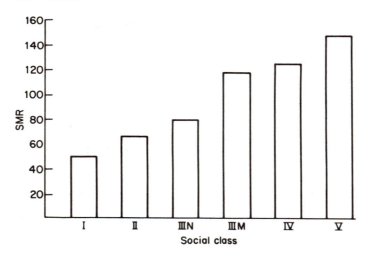

Fig. 4.6   Social class distribution of stomach cancer mortality. SMRs for males aged 15—64. (Data from OPCS.)

mortality rate experienced in their own country. Japanese migrants to Hawaii show rates intermediate between those in Japan and those in the U.S.A.

The average mortality rate for a whole country may hide notable differences in distribution within it. Howe (1970) has demonstrated that, at least in the early 1960s, the standardized mortality ratios for stomach cancer were relatively high in parts of the north of England and in north western Wales. Investigations into this remarkable localization have produced bizarre and inexplicable results. In Caernavonshire, Merioneth and Cheshire, garden soil from properties where people had died from stomach cancer after 15 or more years of residence had higher median concentrations of zinc or chromium than garden soils in the same area where a person had died of a cause other than malignant disease, or had died of cancer after a residence of less than two years. Stocks and Davies (1964) showed that the zinc/copper ratio was consistently higher in the garden soil of houses where persons had died of stomach cancer after ten or more years residence than in gardens of houses where similar persons had died of non-malignant causes. It was also found that the zinc/copper ratio in potatoes grown in such soils correlated well with the soil ratio. In Welsh districts with a relatively high stomach cancer mortality, but not elsewhere, the incidence of stomach cancer after 10—19 years of residence is excessive where the garden has a high content of inorganic carbon, for example in peaty areas.

Chile, Costa Rica and Argentina show relatively high mortality rates from stomach cancer when compared with the rest of the American Continent (see Fig. 4.3). In some cases, for example in Chile, a high dietary intake of nitrates has been identified, usually from the use of nitrogen bearing fertilizers and the consequent contamination of water supplies. N-nitroso compounds (N-nitrosamines and N-nitrosamides) are known, from experiments, to be powerful carcinogens in animals. These compounds can be formed, as a result of digestive processes, in the acid stomach of man, and, hypothetically, they may be formed in relatively high concentration when there is a high dietary intake of inorganic nitrogen. They might then act as a carcinogen on the stomach lining. Tinned and preserved meats and sausages may contain nitrites as preservatives, and are common in the Western diet. However, nitrate and nitrite intakes in the U.K. are considerably lower than those in the populations studied in Chile and Columbia; there is clearly scope for much more research on this particular topic.

4.4.1 Cancer of the colon

Geographical distribution of cancer of the colon tends to show a reciprocal relationship to that of the stomach (cf. Fig. 4.3). Thus, globally, it occurs less commonly in Japan than in the U.S.A. In general terms, cancer of the colon tends to be a disease of industrialized western countries. As a result, one hypothesis which has gained support in recent years is that it is related to the diet consumed in developed countries, and, more specifically, its fibre content. Dietary fibre is made up of a number of compounds each of which may have its own particular effects within the gastrointestinal tract. Methods have been evolved for estimating dietary fibre content quantitatively. Fibre tends to have a laxative effect, holding water and increasing faecal bulk. The amount of fibre in the diet thus determines the volume and consistency of the stool, and also influences the so-called 'transit time', i.e. the time taken for food particles to travel through the digestive system.

The more highly refined diets of modern western societies have a reduced fibre content, and as a result the bowel functions less frequently and sometimes with some difficulty. Researchers have suggested that the increased transit time may be an important factor, allowing the accumulation of products of bacterial metabolism, some of which may be carcinogenic. Again prominent here are the nitrosamines which may result from the breakdown of nitrogenous material.

4.5 Carcinogenesis

The growth of a cell is controlled by the DNA found in its nucleus. DNA comprises the chromosomes which carry the genetic code of the individual. Interference with the structure of the DNA may lead to a mutation, rendering the cell more open to influences destroying its growth control; such a mutation could therefore be carcinogenic in nature. Mutations occurring in the germ cells of the reproductive system are capable of transmission to succeeding generations.

Mutation is one way in which a cell may be primed, as it were, to become a cancer cell. Two fundamental states — usually referred to as *initiation* and *promotion* — are now recognized in the creation of a cancer at cellular level. Some environmental agents may act as initiators, some as promoters, and some as both. After the initiation stage, the cell is a potential cancer cell, waiting only for the 'trigger' stimulus of a promoting agent to effect the final transformation into uncontrolled growth and invasion of surrounding and distant tissues.

Sufficient examples have been given to illustrate ways in which observation of the occurrence of cancer and its association with environmental factors leads to the conclusion that much cancer is determined by environmental influences. Part of this effect may be related to exposure to recognizable and specific agents which are presumably acting as initiators or promoters of the cancer. Since, in many instances, the details of these mechanisms have not been worked out, it may still be unwise to state that a given agent actually 'causes' cancer. However, there is no doubt of the close association between exposure to certain agents and a significantly increased risk of developing cancer. Here, as in so many aspects of medicine and human biology, the remarkable variability in the response of individuals to specific factors plays an important part. It is the group experience which defines the real relative risk; it is not possible to draw valid or even sensible conclusions from anecdotal evidence based on individual experience.

Carcinogens may be considered under the following headings: (*a*) biological agents; (*b*) physical agents; and (*c*) chemical agents, inorganic and organic.

4.5.1   Biological agents (viruses)

Since 1911, when Rous first identified a virus causing tumours in chickens, it has been known that viruses are capable of causing cancer in animals. Since then a number of animal cancers have been found to be attributable to viruses (Table 4.6). Both DNA and RNA type viruses (see Table 3.2) have been implicated, and it is of interest that the DNA viruses are herpes viruses. It is possible to prove that these agents cause cancer in animals by undertaking experiments in transmission of infection from one animal to another. It is more difficult to identify the possible role of viruses in human cancer. There is some circumstantial evidence, although scientific proof is lacking. Transmission experiments are out of the question, the relative longevity of the human species makes the tracing of possible links between cases extremely difficult, and the variability of the biological response complicates the interpretation of the occurrence or non-occurrence of cancer in the presence of infection. If viruses are found in cancer cells they may only be 'passengers', and if they are found more frequently than might be expected, this may simply be because the cancerous cells, being different, are more prone to infection.

Table 4.6   Animal tumours caused by viruses.

Animal	Tumour
Chicken	Sarcoma, leukaemia, lymphoma
Mice	Mammary cancer, leukaemia
Cats	Lymphosarcoma, leukaemia
Frogs	Renal cancer
Monkeys	Lymphoid tumours

One indication that a condition may be due to an infectious agent is the clustering of cases in space and time. Some workers claim to have demonstrated that cases of human leukaemia or of the lymphoid cancer known as Hodgkin's disease tend to cluster in this way, although this is by no means the universal experience.

A herpes virus has been quite definitely associated with a human lymphoma which occurs in African children, and conclusive evidence has been adduced that it is transmitted by mosquitos. The virus has been isolated and characterized by M.A. Epstein and Y.M. Barr and is now known as the E.B. virus. When incubated outside the body with a culture of human lymphocytes the virus brings about changes in the lymphocytes, similar to those seen when cells become malignant, including the development of a more primitive (embryonic) appearance with relatively large nuclei, and a propensity to proliferate continuously — not a usual characteristic of human lymphocytes in culture. Antibodies to the virus are always found in relatively high concentration in patients with Burkitts lymphoma, although they are only present, at much lower levels, in 45 to 50% of unaffected (control) subjects.

E.B. virus is now known to be the cause of infectious mononucleosis (glandular fever) which is a common infection of teenage children. The appearances of the mononuclear white cells of the blood are very similar to those seen in some cases of leukaemia, although in this instance the condition is always self limiting.

The association between genital infection with herpes virus and cancer of the cervix (p. 62) and the way in which this cancer occurs more commonly (although not exclusively) in women who have had multiple sexual encounters, is another set of circumstances which points towards the possible role of viruses in human cancer. In passing, it should be noted that the common wart, which is a benign type of skin growth, is known to be infectious and due to a virus.

4.5.2 Physical agents

Radiation can cause cancer in animals and in man. Radiation also produces mutations, and the two effects are undoubtedly linked. The most penetrating kind of radiation (excluding neutrons, which have to be artificially produced) is gamma radiation. X-rays are similar. Tissues and organs show considerable variability in their sensitivity to radiation. Cells which are actively growing tend to be the most sensitive. Blood cells and cells of blood forming organs are particularly susceptible and often show the earliest effects — leukaemia has been seen as the consequence of irradiation in many studies. Breast cancer, thyroid cancer (especially in women), lung cancer, and cancer of the digestive tract have also been attributed to the effects of radiation. There is considerable uncertainty about the nature of the dose-response relationship in radiation induced cancer; its effects are believed to be cumulative so that prolonged low level exposure might have an equivalent effect to a shorter period of more intense radiation. However, it is not clear whether the relationship between radiation absorbed and cancer risk is of a linear, or more complex, possibly quadratic, nature. Because of the potential effects of relatively low but continuous exposure and the lengthy induction period of cancer, very long follow-up studies of those who have been exposed to radiation are required.

Several investigations have been carried out. An early study of the survivors of the atomic bomb explosions in Japan demonstrated an increased incidence of leukaemia in those who had been most heavily irradiated (Table 4.7). A latent

Table 4.7 Results of irradiation in persons exposed to atomic bomb explosion. (From Maloney, W.C. (1955). *New England Journal of Medicine*, **253**, 88.)

Distance from hypocentre (metres)	Survivors		Rates of leukaemia	
	Severely irradiated	Lightly or not irradiated	Severely irradiated	Lightly or not irradiated
Under 2500	5700	41 900	1:172	1:3223
Over 2500	850	49 650	—	1:12 912

period of several years was noted, similar to that which has been found in experimentally induced leukaemia in mice. The peak incidence of leukaemia occurred in 1959, 14 years after the bombs exploded. Persons exposed to X-radiation for diagnostic or therapeutic purposes have also been studied. Dr Alice Stewart and her colleagues carried out an extensive retrospective investigation of children who developed malignant disease in order to investigate a possible relationship to (*inter alia*) exposure to X-rays. In a controlled study over several years, an increased risk of cancer, especially of leukaemia, was demonstrated in those children who had been irradiated *in utero* because of prenatal X-ray examinations of their mothers. Those children who had been so irradiated had approximately double the risk of dying from cancer before the age of ten years when compared with their non-irradiated contemporaries. The finding was confirmed by an independent study carried out by B. McMahon in the U.S.A. As a result of these findings, doctors now ban X-ray examinations of pregnant women, especially if they involve X-raying the pelvis.

A. Court Brown and R. Doll showed that, amongst over 14 000 patients suffering from ankylosing spondylitis (a painful spinal condition in which the vertebrae of the lower part of the spine become stuck together so that the back becomes stiff) who were treated by X-irradiation during the years 1934 to 1954, there was a ten-fold increase in the occurrence of leukaemia. Children who were treated by X-irradiation for 'enlargement of the thymus gland' subsequently showed an increased propensity to develop thyroid cancer. Women who have had repeated chest X-rays for the surveillance of tuberculosis, and those given X-ray treatment for post-partum mastitis have shown increased rates of breast cancer. It is important to note that in all these studies, with the possible exception of the children who were irradiated *in utero*, moderate to high total doses of radiation were administered. The dose received is not to be compared with the much lower level associated with an occasional chest X-ray for instance.

Nuclear waste in the environment gives rise to levels of exposure very considerably less than those due to medical activities. Only about 0.1% of the average radiation dose to the population of the United Kingdom derives from radioactive waste, and this has to be compared with 70% from natural background and up to 30% from medical procedures. It thus seems highly probable that, in spite of anxiety to the contrary, the health effects of exposure to radioactive waste are commensurately small. Care has, of course, to be taken that radioactive nuclides of the kind found in radioactive waste do not become concentrated in the food chain, or in human tissues. In these circumstances the nuclide radiation could become concentrated in specific tissues or organs, and if persistent, could lead to harmful effects.

Ultraviolet light

In recent years the skin cancer known as malignant melanoma has been showing a significant increase in white races. There is a fair amount of epidemiological evidence that exposure to sunlight may be an important causal factor in the genesis of this condition. Superimposed on the steady increase in incidence noted in Connecticut, U.S.A. has been a succession of waves of increased incidence. Investigators in the University of Connecticut School of Medicine have shown that these relate to periodicity in the activity of the sun — peak sun spot activity, which leads to a decrease in the ability of the stratospheric ozone layer to absorb short wavelength ultraviolet radiation, is followed some 3 to 5 years later by a peak in the incidence of melanoma. In England and Wales, where the steady increase in the incidence of melanomas has also been noted, the rise in the various health regions of the country has been examined in parallel with their experience of sunshine. The rates of increase correlated well with the hours of sunshine recorded in the regions two years earlier. In Norway, the incidence of malignant melanoma has been shown to vary between regions of the country, and to show a threefold difference between north and south with the lower incidence occurring in the northern region where exposure to sunlight is relatively less.

The effects of sunlight on the skin are due to its ultraviolet component. The ultraviolet spectrum is arbitrarily divided into three zones:

Long wavelength	UV-A	320–400 nm
Medium wavelength	UV-B	290–319 nm
Short wavelength	UV-C	less than 290 nm

In general terms, the shorter the wavelength, the more biologically active is the radiation. The short wavelengths are extremely active, and can be used as a bactericidal agent. However, much of the UV-C is filtered out by the ozone layer of the stratosphere, so that very little reaches the earth's surface. There has been some anxiety that the use of long-lived fluorocarbon aerosols and refrigerants could weaken the effect of this natural filter; an increase in skin cancer might then be expected to follow. This conclusion is in line with the observations related to sunspot activity referred to earlier.

The UV-B component of sunlight is largely responsible for the unpleasant effects of sunburn — the delayed erythema (redness of the skin), pain and blistering. It is known that ultraviolet radiation has damaging effects upon the DNA of the epithelial cells, calling for subsequent enzymatic excision and repair. Failure of the repair mechanism could lead to mutations, so that ultraviolet light is potentially mutagenic. Prolonged exposure to sunlight is associated with the condition known as solar keratosis (localized thickening of the skin) there is, of course, the usual variability in susceptibility to these effects. UV-B has caused skin cancer in animal experiments and the results suggest that its carcinogenic effect is cumulative and that the incidence of cancer is directly proportional to the square root of the annual dose.

UV-A is the least active part of the spectrum of ultraviolet light, but is still capable of stimulating the formation of melanin in the skin, so leading to the acquisition of a 'tan'. The burning effect is minimal. Much credence is placed by white races on the value of a skin tan as an indicator of a state of good health. There is no scientific basis for this belief, although phototherapy can be used with benefit to treat certain skin conditions, and there may be a marginal improvement in Vitamin D availablility to the body, especially if the diet is deficient in this respect. A tan without burning may be acquired by using filtered ultraviolet light and solaria utilizing this technique are becoming increasingly popular. Whether the net increase in the exposure of the population to ultraviolet light will be accompanied by any resultant increase in skin cancer remains to be seen. It seems likely that, because the least active part of the ultraviolet spectrum is used, any effect would be so slight as to be undetectable amongst the general background of skin cancers, but not all dermatologists are entirely happy about the indiscriminate use of increasing amounts of ultraviolet.

4.5.3 Chemical agents

Chemicals may act as initiators, promoters, or both, and exhibit all grades of potency. Such complexities, combined with variable induction periods, some of which are remarkably long, add to the difficulties of unravelling the web of causation of cancer. There is more than a million fold difference in the potency of different chemical carcinogens, as can be demonstrated in animal experiments and from human experience. In some instances exposure to small doses over limited periods of time may lead to the development of cancer in a significant proportion of those exposed. At the other end of the scale, exposure of animals to artificially massive doses over relatively long periods may be necessary to induce cancer in just a few, and there may be little or no evidence to substantiate a charge of carcinogenicity in man. It is not always sound to project the results of animal experiments directly to human experience; the definitive proof of carcinogenic activity in man must rely upon the careful accumulation of observations in a planned way and their analysis by undertaking epidemiological studies of relationships between exposure to specific chemicals and the subsequent development of cancer. Such studies are always time consuming and expensive. It is also quite inappropriate to equate the risks of exposure to a potent compound such as aflatoxin, which is known to be capable of producing primary liver cancer in animals and in man, to those of exposure to a substance such as cyclamate, the use of which has been banned in the U.S.A. solely on account of its carcinogenicity in animal experiments. The degree of risk associated with any substance has to be weighed against its value in use and the precautions which can be taken in handling it.

Chemicals causing cancer can be grouped into inorganic or organic substances, and the latter may be further subdivided into those used for industrial purposes, where the hazard is mainly occupational, and those which are biological in nature or used for medical or pharmaceutical purposes. Inorganic chemicals may be minerals, elements or their inorganic compounds.

Minerals and elements

Asbestos consists of six naturally occurring minerals. Crocidolite, amosite, anthophyllite, tremolite and actinolite are all very similar in their crystalline structure, and are compounded with metals. Crocidolite and amosite contain iron, anthophyllite contains magnesium, and tremolite and actinolite contain magnesium and calcium. Chrysotile is fibrous in structure and contains magnesium and silica; it is the most widely distributed form of asbestos and has a wide range of uses in construction and insulation and the production of friction pads such as brake linings. Being fibrous, it is the form of asbestos used in the manufacture of flame proof textiles. Crocidolite is of particular use where resistance to acid is necessary, but its use is now greatly restricted by legislation because of its association with mesothelioma. This hazard has already been described in this chapter, as has also the association of asbestos exposure with lung cancer.

Of the metallic elements, nickel, chromium and their salts are associated with the risk of cancer of the nasal sinuses; iron, as haematite, is associated with lung cancer; and cadmium has been linked with the occurrence of cancer of the prostate.

Organic chemicals

Amongst carcinogens, organic chemicals are represented in much greater numbers than are the inorganic. Perhaps this is because they are more closely related to the chemistry of life, and more readily interact with DNA and other chemical systems of the body. The group of aromatic amines is important, especially in relation to the causation of bladder cancer. Beta-naphthylamine was used for many years in the rubber industry as an antioxidant, but many workers exposed to it have subsequently developed cancer of the bladder; 4-amino-biphenyl, used in dye manufacture, has been similarly incriminated. Other compounds in this group include benzene itself — the parent organic compound from which the others are derived — benzidene, orthodiamisidine, 4-nitro-diphenyl, and orthotolidine. It is believed that these compounds owe their commonality of effect to the end products of their metabolism in the body, and the formation of orthohydroxy amino metabolites.

Nitrosamines have been shown to be carcinogenic in animal experiments, but there is no firm evidence so far of their carcinogenicity in the human, although there is some circumstantial evidence in relation to gastrointestinal cancer. Polychlorinated biphenyls have also come under suspicion because of their carcinogenicity in animals.

Vinyl chloride is used in the plastics industry, when polymerized it forms the widely used material PVC (polyvinyl chloride). The normally rare liver tumour known as angiosarcoma has occurred with very considerably enhanced frequency amongst workers who have handled vinyl chloride — the increase is estimated as about four hundred fold. Chloromethyl ether is used in industry as an ion exchange resin, and in the synthesis of some organic compounds. An excess of lung cancer has been reported amongst workers handling this chemical. Small amounts of bischloromethyl ether are often present as a contaminant; experiments in animals suggest that this is a powerful carcinogen.

Organic compounds are also used as pharmaceuticals, and there is some evidence that on occasions such materials can lead to the occurrence of cancer. Oestrogens given artificially over prolonged periods may increase the risk of developing cancer of the uterus, and a small study in the U.S.A. has shown that administration of diethyl stilboestrol seems to have resulted in an increased incidence of ovarian cancer. The daughters of women who were given stilboestrol during pregnancy have subsequently shown an increased incidence of vaginal cancer. The use of phenacetin as an analgesic has largely discontinued because of the occurrence of kidney damage and occasionally of cancer of the kidney in some of those taking it in large amounts. It is of interest that phenacetin is metabolized to an end product closely similar to those derived from the aromatic hydrocarbons.

The compound chlornaphthazine (N.N.-Bis(2-chloroethyl)-2-naphthylamine) has been used to treat polycythaemia (a disease of the blood in which there is overproduction of red blood cells) and Hodgkins disease, but its use was found to be associated with a rise in the incidence of bladder cancer and it has now gone out of favour. Perhaps this should not have been a great surprise in view of its relationship to beta-naphthylamine.

Injections of iron dextran for the treatment of anaemia have induced cancer in experimental animals, but there is no convincing evidence that cancer has resulted from its use in the human.

4.5.4 Evidence from animal experiments

New substances which may be used as pharmaceuticals or as food additives are tested for carcinogenicity by administering them to animals. Although the results of animal experiments cannot be extrapolated directly to man, especially if the circumstances of the experiment are highly artificial, demonstration of carcinogenicity in animals must lead to some caution in the use of the substances concerned.

When suspicion of this kind has been aroused, it is plainly sensible to take note of the possible risk and to undertake careful observations to discover whether it really exists and, if so, its magnitude. The hazard then has to be weighed against the disbenefits of doing away with it. Life cannot be risk free; a similar judgement is made every time a road is crossed. There are degrees of risk; the potential carcinogenicity has to be weighed against its value in use. On this kind of consideration, it might be thought that it is more important to stop smoking cigarettes than to stop using saccharin, which has come under suspicion solely because it seems to have the potential of causing bladder cancer in rats if it is administered to them in massive doses; there is absolutely no evidence to link the use of saccharine with human bladder cancer.

5
Coronary heart disease

5.1 The importance of coronary heart disease

Each year, in England and Wales, nearly 600 000 deaths occur. A little over half of them are due to disease affecting the heart or blood vessels (Fig. 5.1).

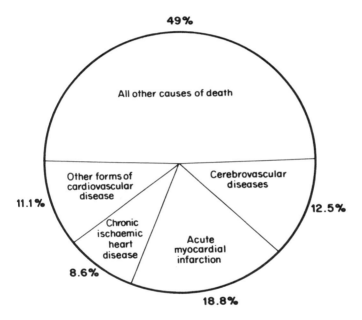

Fig. 5.1 Cardiovascular diseases as causes of mortality. Circulatory diseases cause more than half of all deaths in England and Wales. Of the main subdivisions, ischaemic heart disease causes the largest proportion. Acute myocardial infarction is the biggest segment of ischaemic heart disease, and causes 18.8% of all deaths. (Based on OPCS mortality statistics for 1978.)

Those deaths falling within the general category of the circulatory system may be further subdivided, the main subgroups being hypertension, ischaemic heart disease of the coronary arteries, disease of the blood vessels supplying the brain (cerebrovascular disease) and all other diseases affecting the arteries, veins and lymphatics. Deaths from ischaemic heart disease may occur very suddenly (acute myocardial infarction, see p. 81) and account for 36% of all deaths from circulatory disease or 18.8% of all deaths. Chronic ischaemic heart disease is a more slowly developing form of the condition, which may be accompanied by recurrent chest pain, or may be present as a progressive slide into heart failure; this form particularly affects older age groups.

Although ischaemic heart disease is a most important cause of mortality in the U.K., it does not show up as a particularly prominent cause of morbidity since, particularly in general practice, but also in hospital medicine, it is submerged by a mass of less important and non-fatal conditions. Information about its occurrence in general practice can be obtained from analysis of sickness benefit claims or from special surveys of attendances at general practitioners' surgeries. Sickness certificates mentioning ischaemic heart disease constitute less than 2% of all sickness benefit claims, but in any case these only cover those persons of working age. Table 5.1 gives an analysis of patients attending general practitioner surgeries, and demonstrates the variation with increasing age. As far as hospital medicine is

Table 5.1   General practitioners' patients consulting for conditions due to ischaemic heart disease as a percentage of those consulting for all conditions (from OPCS, 1974).

Age groups	All conditions		Acute myocardial infarction		Angina of effort		Other ischaemic heart disease	
	No.	(100%)	No.	(%)	No.	(%)	No.	(%)
0– 4	19370		—	—	—	—	1	—
5–14	30766		1	--	2	—	2	—
15–24	29407		2	—	3	—	1	—
25–44	48942		55	(0.1)	42	(0.1)	47	(0.1)
45–64	43608		477	(1.1)	536	(1.2)	535	(1.2)
65–74	14688		284	(1.9)	425	(2.9)	509	(3.5)
75–	9511		177	(1.9)	232	(2.4)	461	(4.9)
All	196292		996	(0.5)	1240	(0.6)	1556	(0.8)

concerned, information is available from the hospital inpatient survey or from Hospital Activity Analysis. Table 5.2 demonstrates the discharge rates per 10 000 population for all diseases, and for the main categories of cardiovascular disease. Such figures cannot include many of those persons who die suddenly as a result of acute myocardial infarction without any previous evidence of sickness.

Disease of the coronary arteries is more common in men. In both sexes the death rates increase with increasing age, and female rates approach those of males in the older age groups (Fig. 5.2). Other forms of vascular disease are less common causes of mortality, but atherosclerosis (hardening of the arteries) affecting the blood vessels of the brain makes an important contribution, accounting for 12% of total mortality in England and Wales.

This pattern of cardiovascular disease is found particularly in industrially developed or developing countries. It contrasts with the situation in poorer societies, where infectious and parasitic diseases such as tuberculosis, malaria and gastroenteritis are frequently the major causes of death. Such diseases, particularly tuberculosis, were major scourges in Western countries in the recent past, although they have now given way to the relative predominance of cardiovascular disease.

Table 5.2 Discharge rates age 15 years and over per 10 000 population by age and sex (M = male, F = female). (From Hospital Inpatient Enquiry, D.H.S.S., 1975.)

		All ages	15–	20–	25–	35–	45–	65–	75+
All causes	M	830.2	505.2	513.4	453.0	510.0	895.6	1625.1	2639.7
	F	1156.0	1152.4	2234.8	1932.1	965.2	793.6	1121.8	1964.8
Acute myocardial infarction	M	25.9	–	0.1	1.5	12.2	58.6	92.9	93.9
	F	11.6	–	0.1	0.3	2.0	14.2	42.3	55.4
Other ischaemic heart disease	M	12.2	–	0.1	0.8	8.1	28.2	35.9	49.2
	F	7.4	–	–	0.4	2.6	10.6	21.2	36.2
Rheumatic heart disease	M	2.9	0.4	0.8	0.9	3.3	7.4	5.1	2.8
	F	4.1	0.6	0.8	1.4	5.5	9.2	6.7	4.4
Hypertensive disease	M	4.5	0.4	0.8	1.3	4.5	10.5	12.6	7.5
	F	4.6	0.6	2.2	2.6	3.8	7.5	11.2	11.4
Other forms of heart disease	M	19.8	1.3	2.0	2.8	5.5	25.1	80.0	184.2
	F	28.6	0.7	0.8	1.7	4.1	13.1	48.1	141.2

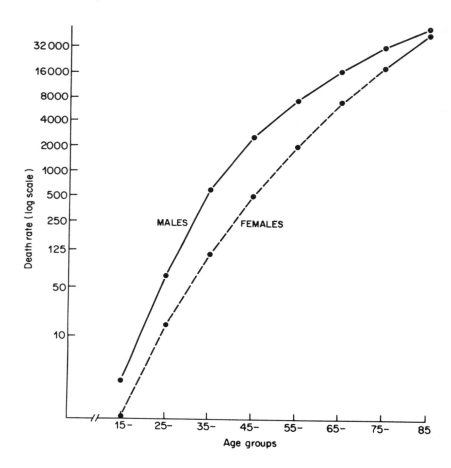

Fig. 5.2   Ischaemic heart disease (ICCD 410–414). Death rates per million living, by age and sex. (Data from OPCS.)

An epidemic may be described as an increase in the occurrence of a disease with the passage of time to such an extent that it significantly exceeds the average for previous years. It is important to realise that the time-space scale is relative. It is not difficult to recognize an epidemic of, say, typhoid fever which builds up over a period of two or three weeks in a single locality. However, if an outbreak is less confined in space and time it is not usually immediately recognizable — for instance, since the cases of congenital deformities associated with the use of thalidomide in the 1960s were occurring in numerous scattered locations the increase was not recognized for several months, by which time over 800 children in the U.K. alone were affected.

Mortality from disease of the coronary arteries has been increasing in the United Kingdom, as, indeed in many other countries, but it took several years for the epidemic nature of the increase to be appreciated. As this happened, during the late twenties and thirties and beyond, so the classification of the condition in the

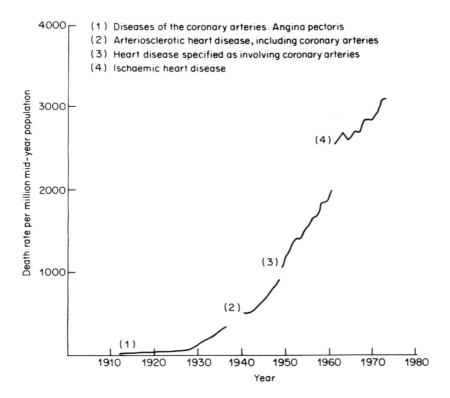

Fig. 5.3 Trends in coronary heart disease mortality in England and Wales, 1910–75. (Data from Registrar General Statistical Reviews (various years) and OPCS.)

International Classification of Causes of Death (ICCD) became progressively more refined (see p. 5).

Figure 5.3 demonstrates this upturn in mortality, which appears to have started in the mid to late 1920s. The problem of changing definitions in successive classifications makes it impossible to plot a continuous line but, whichever definition is considered, it is plain that death from coronary disease was diagnosed comparatively very much less frequently in the earlier years of this century than it is today. Some have attempted to argue that much of this increase is spurious. Coronary disease is seen mostly in older persons – the proportion of elderly in our population has increased. Doctors have become more aware of the condition – therefore are more likely to ascribe death to it. Diagnosis has become more accurate – therefore death from coronary artery disease is more frequently recognized. Most of these arguments do not stand up to critical examination. For example, that about the increasing proportion of the elderly in the population is largely dispelled when age specific rates are examined (Fig. 5.4). Indeed, coronary disease is an important cause of premature mortality, and when it occurs in relatively younger men, is particularly prone to lead to sudden death, with little or no warning. This must give rise to considerable concern, for these are men who are approaching the

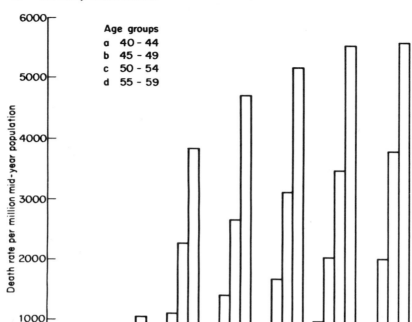

Fig. 5.4   Trends in age specific death rates per million for coronary heart disease. Males aged 40 to 59 in England and Wales, 1931–75. (Data from Registrar General Statistical Reviews (various years) and OPCS.)

height of their responsibilities, often with young and dependent families and holding jobs in which their maturity and experience are important attributes. Sudden death in such circumstances represents a catastrophe of major proportions for the family, with potentially severe social and emotional consequences, while the economist would point to the importance of this particular group of men to the national economy. There is no doubt that coronary artery disease is a problem of major importance in the United Kingdom, and that, if it is possible to identify and modify environmental factors which are associated with its occurrence, no effort should be spared so to do.

5.2   The nature of coronary heart disease

The coronary arteries are comparatively small vessels which run down the front and back of the heart conveying a blood supply from the main artery of the body (the aorta) to the heart muscle. If a coronary artery, or one of its branches, becomes obstructed the related area of heart muscle will be starved of oxygen and other essential nutrients because of the reduced blood supply. The muscle will be weakened and some of the cells will die. If the affected individual exerts himself, the oxygen deprived muscle will ache, leading to the chest pain known as angina. Such deprivation of the heart muscle's blood supply is known as myocardial ischaemia; once established, it may become progressively worse with advancing age. Total obstruction of a coronary artery may occur suddenly if the blood clots in an already partially obstructed vessel (coronary thrombosis). Such an event must lead inevitably to the total death of the patch of heart muscle supplied by the obstructed artery (myocardial infarction) and this event frequently results in sudden cessation of the heart's action and the immediate death of the individual.

The common cause of the initial narrowing of the coronary arteries is a condition known as atheroma, characterized by the occurrence of small localized swellings just under the inner lining of the vessels. The swellings project into the lumen of the artery and so narrow it. Such deposits also occur in larger arteries, especially the aorta, but in such large vessels do not lead to significant obstruction. The deposits consist of localized accumulations of fatty fibrous tissue associated with the deposition of cholesterol from the blood. This deposition is very important in the causation of vascular disease and has been the subject of much investigation. In modern industrialized and relatively affluent societies it appears to commence quite early in life and the resulting atheroma becomes increasingly extensive with increasing age. Even in relatively young male adults significant degrees of the condition may be found, as evidenced by a number of studies. Table 5.3 summarizes the results of a study carried out by postmortem examination of the coronary

Table 5.3 Results of necropsy studies of coronary arteries of fit British males killed in flying accidents. (From Mason, J.K. (1963). *British Medical Journal, 2, 1234.*)

Age group	Percentage showing	
	macroscopic disease	more than 50% occlusion
17–24	14.1	5.1
25–33	35.9	19.1
34–42	62.5	50.0

arteries of a series of British males aged between 17 and 42 years, all of whom were victims of flying accidents, and all of whom were graded as physically fit before they met their deaths. The mean age of the group was 27.3 years. 'Significant luminal restriction of one or more coronary arteries' was demonstrated in 21.9% of cases. Another study of 300 American soldiers, with an average age of 22.1 years, who were killed in the Korean war showed that in 12.3% at least one of the main coronary arteries was narrowed by atheroma to half or less of its original lumen (Enos, Holmes and Beyer, 1953).

5.3 Genetic influences

Genetic factors undoubtedly play their part in the development of atheroma. In the disease known as familial hypercholesterolaemia an inherited tendency to a raised level of cholesterol in the blood serum is accompanied by an enhanced risk of suffering from coronary disease. Diabetics are also more prone to coronary disease, and diabetes has an important genetic component. Carefully conducted comparative studies have demonstrated that persons who have a first degree relative who has died from coronary disease have a greater risk of developing it than those without such relatives. In one study men under the age of 55 who had a male relative who had died of the condition under the age of 55 experienced a five fold increase in risk. The corresponding factor in women was 2.5 (Slack and Evans, 1966).

5.4   Nutritional factors

The genetic background is only part of the picture, for a variety of environmental factors have been shown to influence the risk of developing coronary atheroma. The first point to note has already been mentioned — the disease is one which tends to become more important and more common in relatively affluent societies. Thus in Britain, improving social conditions have been accompanied by an increasing incidence of coronary disease, a point to which we shall return later (p. 85). International differences in the occurrence of the condition are easily identified by mortality information published by the World Health Organization (W.H.O.), although there are some constraints on making comparisons between different countries due to varying standards of diagnosis and certification and registration of death. Information is available to W.H.O. for some 65 countries: relative mortality from ischaemic heart disease is highest in Finland, South Africa, the U.S.A., Scotland, Australia, Northern Ireland, New Zealand, Canada, Iceland and Israel; death rates are consistently low in Thailand, Honduras, Guatemala, El Salvador, Taiwan, Ecuador, Paraguay, Jordan, Peru, the Phillipines, and Hong Kong; and death rates are rising in Czechoslavakia, France, Netherlands and England and Wales.

Studies have demonstrated that populations with relatively high levels of serum cholesterol and lipo-proteins circulating in the blood have an increased incidence of atheroma and a correspondingly increased risk of coronary heart disease. There has, therefore, been very considerable interest in the factors which can be shown to influence serum cholesterol levels, and a great deal of research has been carried out.

During the 1940s Keys and his co-workers showed that populations with a relatively high dietary fat intake tended to have the higher cholesterol levels which appear to be associated with coronary atheroma. Further studies have suggested that it is not only the quantity but also the quality of the dietary fat which is important. Diets containing a high proportion of animal fat appear to be more atherogenic than those with a more equitable admixture of the polyunsaturated fats derived from vegetable or fish sources. The relationships between standards of living, nutritional status, proportions of saturated and unsaturated fats in the diet and serum cholesterol levels were well demonstrated in studies carried out by Bronte-Stewart, Keys and Brook in a single area in Cape Province, South Africa. They examined three separate ethnic and socially different groups, but since they all lived in the same area, any geographical or geological factors which might have affected studies comparing groups living in different countries were eliminated, and the methods used in the study could also be standardized. The groups studied were the very poor Bantu, the Cape coloured population, who were better off than the Bantu but not so well off as the third group, the affluent Europeans. This study showed that, as the standard of living improved, so did the total amount of fat in the diet and the proportion of saturated animal fat to unsaturated vegetable fat (Fig. 5.5). The β-lipid content of the blood serum, which contains the cholesterol component, was highest in the Europeans, intermediate in the Cape coloureds, and lowest in the Bantu, and thus was directly correlated with their standards of living and the fat contents of their diets.

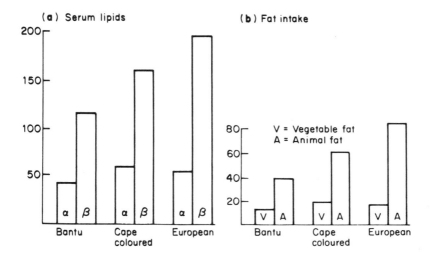

Fig. 5.5 (a) Serum lipid levels and (b) fat intake for populations in Cape Province. (From Bronte-Stewart *et al.*, 1955.)

Naturally, as a result of such studies, attempts have been made to reduce the risk of developing coronary thrombosis by giving diets containing high levels of unsaturated fats. These trials have not been very successful, but perhaps this is not surprising, since it would appear to be the diet consumed from quite an early age which determines the degree of atheroma in the arteries. However, long term trials in apparently well people, using drugs to lower serum cholesterol, have met with some success, the main effect appearing to be a reduction of the incidence of acute episodes in persons suffering from angina.

Attention has also been turned towards the carbohydrate content of diet, and particularly the effects of refining carbohydrates. Yudkin (1964) has advocated the hypothesis that the increased incidence of coronary heart disease is associated with an increased intake of carbohydrates, and in one study reported that patients with atherosclerotic disease (but not necessarily coronary disease) tended to have a higher sugar intake than those not so affected. This study has been repeated by others, who failed to confirm it. A great deal of correspondence followed in the medical press. However, Yudkin's theories are to some extent parallel with those of D.P. Burkitt and others in relation to the excessive refinement of roughage in our diet. The refining of sugar, for instance, leads to the removal of all the natural vegetable fibres, and the natural limiting effect upon intake which would be caused by the sheer bulk of the food is thus lost. Yudkin has pointed out that to consume the equivalent of the average day's sugar intake, it would be necessary to eat 1.1 kg

(2½ lbs) of sugar beet. Similar comments can be made about highly refined flour. The higher carbohydrate content consequent upon the reduced fibre of the diet in such circumstances facilitates excessive carbohydrate intake and a propensity to become overweight, if not frankly obese. Excess weight is known to carry with it an increased risk of raised blood pressure, which in its turn is associated with an increased risk of developing coronary heart disease.

There is thus much evidence that the less refined, more vegetable oriented diet which is usually associated with the less affluent standards of life is a healthier diet as far as the avoidance of atheroma and coronary heart disease is concerned. Mankind has, of course, evolved on such a diet, and it is only the increased sophistication of food-stuff handling and preparation, and the higher incomes which have enabled the consumption of greater proportions of animal products, which have led to recent changes. These changes make it too easy to eat in an unbalanced way to which our bodies are not adequately adapted. The old proverb must be changed; enough is *better than* a feast.

5.5   The relevance of exercise

Our modern way of life has also brought about a tremendous change in our methods of work and of movement from place to place, and this also has had its effect on health. The heart is a specialized muscle. It is well recognized that regular exercise of any muscle leads to an increase in its bulk and strength and, in parallel with this, an opening up of extra vascular channels, so increasing its potential blood supply. Conversely, under-used muscles become weak, flabby and inefficient. The heart is exercised by pumping blood around the circulation; if it is regularly made to work fairly vigorously, its strength, bulk, blood supply and efficiency will be at an optimum. On the other hand, the heart of anyone who leads a physically inactive life will inevitably have much less reserve capacity. In particular, individuals whose hearts have a relatively efficient blood supply will be protected to a degree against the effects of incipient or sudden obstruction of one of the channels of supply, since there will be a reserve of other channels which can be used. It might be expected, therefore, that regular exercise, enough to make some demand upon the heart, will protect against coronary disease and that a sedentary mode of life will lead to increased vulnerability to coronary atheroma. This hypothesis has been borne out by studies which show that more active persons tend to have a lower incidence of coronary thrombosis. The classical study was that carried out by Morris on 'bus crews, which showed that conductors had a lower incidence of coronary thrombosis than the drivers (Morris *et al*. 1953). The sedentary work of the drivers contrasted with the continual activity of the conductors both on the level and up and down stairs. Other factors might be playing a part, however, in this case. Morris pointed out that, taken as a group, the drivers tended to have larger body frames and to be heavier than the conductors. There may, therefore, have been some hidden selection which was picking out relatively more overweight, and thus relatively more at risk men as drivers.

Studies have demonstrated that driving itself puts additional strain on the cardiovascular system — physiological changes occur; both blood pressure and heart rate are elevated, especially in difficult traffic conditions. Such changes have also been observed in racing drivers, whose heart rates are considerably increased just before the start of a race. The changes are caused by increased levels of circulating hormones known as catecholamines which are secreted as part of the body's physiological preparedness for action. This is associated with the primitive 'fight or flight' response to a challenge. The response is clearly designed to lead to considerable physical activity but, in the case of the car driver this cannot occur. Advanced modern technology, with its techniques of high speed mechanical transport over long distances thus imposes stresses upon the human organism to which it does not adapt well. The opportunities for active physical exercise which should be associated with transporting ourselves from place to place are lost, and at the same time physiological changes are induced in drivers, mobilizing resources which, in the event, are not required.

5.6   Cigarette smoking

Studies which commenced before the second world war, and which continued at an accelerating pace in the 1940s, 50s and 60s have amply demonstrated the very considerable harm which is done to the collective health of the nation by the smoking of cigarettes. This is a new cultural practice acquired in Europe only during the last hundred years (see Fig. 8.4). In England, it preceded the rise in the incidence of coronary heart disease by only some thirty years. Early investigations showed that those who were classified as having a relatively heavy consumption of cigarettes (20 or more a day) had higher death rates, age for age, than those who were non-smokers. Carefully conducted follow up studies involving many thousands of individuals enabled a more detailed examination of the occurrence of various fatal conditions amongst smokers; one of these was coronary heart disease. The report *Smoking and Health Now* published in 1971 by the Royal College of Physicians cites four important studies, each of which demonstrated that the risk of dying from coronary heart disease was greater amongst cigarette smokers than amongst non-smokers or cigar or pipe smokers. The effect is most noticeable amongst the younger age groups where the risk is two or three times greater than that of non-smokers of corresponding age. The risk factor decreases to about one and a half in older age groups. Cigarette smoking thus emerges as a most important environmental factor, introduced by man himself, which is associated with increased susceptibility to a major cause of premature death in the United Kingdom.

5.7   Effects of social change

It is both interesting and instructive to trace changes in the social class incidence of coronary heart disease since it began to rise in the early part of this century. Social class distributions of mortality can be worked out around the years in which national censuses are held. As part of the census, counts are made of the numbers of persons working in various occupations. Since the occupation of the deceased is recorded when a death is registered the OPCS is able to relate deaths to occupational groups and thus to social class categories. The results are published as decennial reports on occupational mortality. When the rise in the incidence of heart disease was first recognized, it was seen to be occurring predominantly in social class I. This was pointed out in the commentary in the decennial supplement on occupational mortality for the period 1930—32. This early observation was a powerful factor in the growth of the hypothesis that stress predisposed to the risk of developing the condition. Social class I comprises professionals who carry heavy responsibilities and frequently have to solve difficult and intractable problems as part of their daily work. However, it is likely that other social classes were exposed to equally great, though different stresses, especially in the economic climate of the time.

The supplement for the years 1949—53, centred on the census of 1951, carried a comparison of the social class gradients at that time and in the period around 1931. Twenty years after the first rise in coronary disease had been first noted the social class gradient in the standardized mortality ratios upwards from class V to class I was still unmistakeable, although the gradient was less than before. By this time there had been a considerable rise in the mortality rates attributable to coronary heart disease in all social classes. When the male social class mortality was examined by age group, interesting differences emerged. The ratios showed no particular trend in men aged from 20—24, but at 25—34 they indicated an upward mortality gradient from class I to class V. This contrasted with strong downward gradients from I to V at 45—54 and 55—64 (see Table 5.4). It was also noticeable at this time that, when the overall mortality ratios (at ages 20—64) for the periods 1920—32 and 1949—53 were compared, although there was a downward gradient in mortality from social class I to social class V in both periods the gradient was considerably steeper, for men, in the former period. For married women, who gave no evidence of any clear trend in social class mortality in 1949—1953, a downward gradient, similar to that in men, had been in evidence in 1930—1932. Thus, by the time of the 1951 census, there was evidence of a levelling out of the social class differences in coronary disease mortality. Furthermore, although the older men, born before 1907, suffered higher mortality rates in social class I, the younger age groups appeared to show the reverse, although there would, of course, be fewer deaths amongst them.

A more dramatic change was in store ten years later. The figures published for the period around 1961 demonstrated that the greatest mortality now lay in social class V for men and married women aged 20 to 64. The latest available figures, from the decennial supplement on occupational mortality for the period 1970—72 (Table 5.5) show little difference from those of ten years before.

These changes have occurred in parallel with considerable social changes in the UK. By 1951, the Beveridge Report had come and gone, social welfare measures were getting under way, and as a result, a certain amount of social levelling up in standards of nutrition had occurred, aided by the introduction of a national food

Table 5.4   Standardized mortality ratios attributed to angina pectoris and coronary disease in men (M) and married women (F) in England and Wales, 1931 to 1961 by social class. (OPCS data.)

Year (age group)	Social class									
	I		II		III		IV		V	
	M	F	M	F	M	F	M	F	M	F
1931 (35—64)	237	157	148	126	95	93	66	84	67	89
1951 (20—64)	147	102	110	96	105	101	79	104	89	105
1961	98	69	95	81	106	103	96	107	112	143

Table 5.5 Standardized mortality ratios for men aged 15–64 years by social class, England and Wales, 1970–72 (from OPCS, 1978).

Cause of death	Social class					
	I	II	IIIN	IIIM	IV	V
Acute myocardial infarction	88	92	115	107	108	108
Ischaemic heart disease	88	91	114	107	108	111
Chronic ischaemic heart disease	87	86	108	106	111	123

policy during the war. This process has continued and the marked differences between the incomes and living conditions of the various social subsections of the community have been considerably eroded by comparison with the 1930s (Townsend, 1979). At the same time the general standards of living of the whole population have improved. Poverty is relative, and the living standards of those below the poverty line in modern times in this country are higher than those of the poor of sixty years ago — no longer do we see unshod ragamuffins begging for sustenance in our city streets. There can be few who now do not receive an adequate diet, although research indicates that it is the quality and content of diet which is important. The sedentary life has grown apace, with good access to public transport (at least until recent years), many households owning their own cars, and the invention and acquisition of home based entertainments such as radios, music centres, and television. These facilities are available to all classes of society, and few households do not have them.

As the evidence associating an enhanced risk of mortality with the consumption of cigarettes has become more widely known and accepted, changes have been occurring in the smoking habits of the population, but some groups have given up smoking more readily than others. In parallel, their risk of developing and dying from coronary disease has fallen. This is well illustrated by the experience of British doctors, whose smoking habits and mortality experience have been carefully monitored by Sir Richard Doll. Information on his observations is given in the Royal College of Physicians report *Smoking and Health Now*. Between 1953–57 and 1961–65 a 6% fall in coronary disease mortality was recorded in doctors, while in all men in England and Wales there was an apparent 32% increase. Although part of this difference could have been due to differences in the precision of diagnosis in the general public, adjustment for this possible statistical complication only makes a moderate inroad into the difference. This change in the coronary disease experience of doctors accompanied a dramatic change in their smoking habits as many ceased to smoke cigarettes in response to the increasing knowledge of their harmful effects.

The change in doctors' smoking habits has been part of a marked reduction in the smoking of cigarettes by social classes I and II, so that there is now an upward gradient in the quantity of tobacco smoked as cigarettes from social class I to social class V. This may well be an important factor in the reversal of the social class gradient of coronary heart disease mortality which has been noted (p. 85).

As other significant factors in living standards have levelled out the comparative risk has equalized but in addition, because of their greater response to information about the risks of smoking cigarettes, social classes I and II have reaped the additional benefits of giving up the cigarette. As their mortality has stabilized, or even decreased, it has been overtaken by that of other groups in the community, now equally exposed to other factors.

In a recent report in the D.H.S.S. publication *Health Trends* (1981), Marmot and others have also examined these changes in social class distribution. Whilst remarking that there may have been changing emphases in the diagnosis of different forms of heart disease in the social classes they conclude that cigarette smoking and the consumption of relatively more sugar and relatively less wholemeal bread by social classes IV and V may well be associated with the observed changes in incidence.

A pattern of rapid environmental change during the past seventy to one hundred years is thus found to be associated with the change in coronary heart disease mortality. The fat content of our diet has increased, particularly animal fat. The cigarette has established itself. The sedentary way of life has increased apace; during the day we drive around in our cars or lorries, or are transported in buses and trains. Many of us spend our working day sitting at an office desk. In the evenings we sit steadfastly watching our colour television sets. No longer are such activities (or inactivities) the prerogative of the rich. Concurrently with these changes in our environment, we have seen the rise of coronary atheroma as a major cause of ill-health and death, although at a different rate in social subsections of the community where the environmental changes have been able to exert their influence at different times. There is a great deal of evidence to support the view that these various events are closely associated, and that the occurrence of coronary disease could be reduced if we were able to make some adjustments to the ways in which we feed, work, and enjoy our leisure time.

5.8   Water supply and the 'water factor'

There is one other rather mysterious environmental factor which has an unexplained association with the elevated mortality rates from circulatory disease. This is the softness of the water supply. Studies from several different parts of the world indicate that a hard water supply has a protective effect. It has also been shown in the U.K. that deliberate softening of the water supply in some areas has been accompanied by an increase in death rates from circulatory disease. It is to be noted that all circulatory disease appears to be affected by the 'water factor', although the predominant form in any given country shows the major effect. Thus, in Japan, where cerebrovascular disease is the prominent variety of cardiovascular disease it is that which is most affected. In the United Kingdom, therefore, coronary heart disease is particularly noticeably affected. The mechanism of the association is a mystery, although some workers have suggested that the calcium content of the water supply is most likely to be the significant factor. However, since the hardness of the water supply is an effect of the terrain from which it is collected, here is a clear link between the geological environment and the health of the population which is related to it.

6
The lungs

6.1   Anatomy and defences

The trachea in man is approximately 10 to 11 cm long and 2 cm in mean diameter. It is supported by bands of cartilage, and at its lower end divides into two main bronchi, right and left, one to each lung. The main bronchi themselves divide into smaller bronchi up to a total of eleven branchings, the resulting tubes becoming steadily smaller as the process of division occurs. From the twelfth to the sixteenth divisions they are known as bronchioles, continuing to become still smaller as they divide. At the end of this stage they are tiny tubes which, after several more divisions lead to the alveolar ducts, alveolar sacs, and the alveoli themselves. Alveoli are minute cavities with thin delicate walls containing capillary blood vessels, and lined with a single layer of cells through which gaseous diffusion between the air in the alveolus and the blood cells in the capillaries can easily occur. The ultimate area presented to the inspired air by the walls of the hundreds of millions of alveoli in each lung amounts in all to between 70 and 90 square metres.

Air entering the respiratory passages is filtered by hairs and mucus in the nose. The trachea and larger bronchi are lined by a layer of cells each of which bears a minute hair or cilium which is capable of movement. The cilia beat with a constant and coordinated motion, rather as the stalks of corn in a field move synchronously as gusts of wind pass across them. Glands embedded in the walls of the trachea and bronchi produce a film of sticky mucus which lies on and around the cilia and is constantly carried upwards by their coordinated beating movement. Thus is created a remarkable self-cleansing mechanism — a 'ciliary escalator' — constantly trapping fine particles which escape the nasal filter and enter the airways and carrying them up and out of the respiratory tract. The mucus is either swalled or expectorated. As the inspired air passes down the trachea during inhalation a vortex is created which tends to throw particles centrifugally so that they fall upon and are entrapped by the upward gliding film of mucus.

6.2   The fate of inhaled particles

Dust, fumes and smoke contain particles which are capable of penetrating into the lung tissues. Dust particles range in size from a diameter of 1 μm to about 150 μm, whereas those in fumes range between 0.2 and 1 μm. Industrial fumes often consist of oxides formed from hot or burning metals. Smoke has particles of less than 0.3 μm in diameter. Tobacco smoke is a 'wet' smoke, composed of tiny droplets of tar, the particle size being about 0.25 μm. These definitions should not be taken as dogmatic statements, but rather as a general indication of the relative sizes of the particles concerned. Normally only particles less than about 10 μm in diameter will float in air for any length of time, and it is those less than 5 μm in diameter which are likely to penetrate the defences of the lungs and reach the bronchioles and alveoli.

Bacteria and viruses are well within the limits allowing penetration of the respiratory tract. Those which enter the lungs are usually destroyed by the normal protective mechanisms described above and in Chap. 3. However, any accumulation of debris or liquid in the lungs is likely to provide a focus for the growth of opportunistic invaders. Thus local tissue damage or obstruction of the normal airflow or failure to adequately drain the lung of secretions is liable to encourage the development of localized infections. These may then lead to further tissue damage or destruction, so that a vicious circle of recurrent infection and damage is set up. A severe chest infection secondary to an acute illness such as whooping cough or measles, or acute bronchitis following upon a cold may be the initial trigger of this process. In other circumstances the lung may be damaged by allergic processes such as those which occur in asthma, or foreign materials obtaining entry to the bronchioles or alveoli may cause damage which predisposes to subsequent infection.

Respiratory diseases are amongst the three most important groups of diseases contributing to mortality in the United Kingdom; only diseases of the circulatory system and cancer cause greater numbers of deaths each year. Between them, these three groups of disease accounted for almost 87% of mortality in 1979 (Table 6.1).

Table 6.1   Main causes of mortality in England and Wales, 1979 (OPCS data).

Cause of death	Number of deaths	Per cent	
Heart and circulatory disease (including cerebrovascular disease)	298 436	50.3	
Cancer	121 198	21.8	86.6
Respiratory diseases	85 925	14.5	
All diseases	593 019	100.0	

Table 6.2 examines mortality from respiratory disease in greater detail. The relative importance of pneumonia and bronchopneumonia arises from the tendency for intercurrent infection of the lungs, often by opportunistic bacteria, to occur as a terminal event which is recorded as the eventual cause of death. As a result, deaths from these conditions tend to occur more commonly at either end of the age scale (Fig. 6.1).

6.3   Chronic bronchitis

Chronic bronchitis is another common cause of death, but in this case stands on its own as an illness which may persist for many years, leading in some cases to an ever-increasing disability as it progresses. It is characterized by excessive production of mucus by the bronchial glands. Impairment of the drainage of bronchi and bronchioles is accompanied by recurrent bouts of chest infection and consequent damage to and fibrosis of lung tissues. In its more advanced forms, alveolar destruction and scarring lead to the development of small cavities (emphysema), and

Table 6.2   Mortality from respiratory diseases in England and Wales, 1979 (OPCS data).

ICCD no.	Disease		Numbers of deaths
460–519	All respiratory diseases	M	44 024
		F	41 901
480–487	Pneumonia and influenza	M	22 851
		F	32 363
485	Bronchopneumonia	M	20 159
	(organism unspecified)	F	29 741
491	Chronic bronchitis	M	14 540
		F	4 966
500–508	Pneumonoconiosis and other	M	423
	lung disease due to external agents	F	91
500	Coalworkers pneumoconiosis	M	243
		F	—
501	Asbestosis	M	24
		F	5
502	Pneumoconiosis due to other	M	39
	silica or silicates	F	2
503	Pneumoconiosis due to	M	1
	other inorganic dust	F	9
504	Pneumopathy due to	M	9
	inhalation of other dust	F	15
505	Pneumoconiosis	M	56
	(unspecified)	F	—

obstruction of blood flow through the capillaries and other small blood vessels in the lungs. Increased resistance to blood flow through the lungs puts additional strain on the right ventricle of the heart and may eventually lead to heart failure.

Chronic bronchitis is a disease to which residents of the British Isles are particularly prone (Fig. 6.2), and as a result it has been called the 'English disease'. It is an enigmatic condition — Why are males so much more prone to it than females? Is there an inherent constitutional predisposition to develop bronchitis in some people? Why is it particularly prevalent in the British Isles? Much is still unclear, but two particular environmental factors have been found to have an effect on its occurrence. These are atmospheric pollution and cigarette smoking.

It has been recognized for many years that chronic bronchitis occurs more commonly in towns than in country districts. Howe (1970) has illustrated the differences between SMRs in town and country in the U.K. His maps, based on observations made over the period 1954–58, show high SMRs in the northwestern conurbations, in the midland towns in and around Birmingham, in South Wales, and in London and its environs, especially northeast London. On the other hand, low SMRs occurred in counties such as Norfolk, Wiltshire and Cornwall; Devon, Somerset, Dorset, Oxfordshire, Northamptonshire and the central counties of Wales all had SMRs below 100. This distribution still applies. Figures for 1978, relating to the standard regions of England and Wales, as defined by OPCS, are given in Table 6.3.

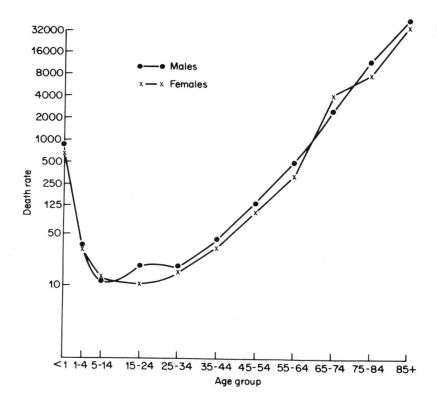

Fig. 6.1   Pneumonia. Death rates per million living by age and sex (Data from OPCS.)

There is much evidence that air pollution is an important factor associated with this distribution. Its potentially damaging effect is demonstrable from an early age. Studies in children have been carried out over a prolonged period and reported in the *British Journal of Preventive and Social Medicine*. A cohort of 4592 children, living in various parts of the country, were followed up since their birth in the first week of March 1946 to 1961 when they were 15 years old. As a substitute for direct measurement of atmospheric pollution levels, which would have been impracticable, local levels of consumption of domestic coal were used to define areas of low, medium, moderate and high pollution. Information about the occurrence of illness was obtained by health visitor interview and special medical examinations were carried out by school medical officers at 6, 7, 11 and 15 years of age. Although there was no statistically significant difference in the occurrence of upper respiratory tract infection according to the type of area in which the children lived, there were very definite and significant differences in the occurrence of *lower* respiratory tract infections such as bronchitis and pneumonia during the early years of life. During the first two years of life there was a steady gradient of morbidity from relatively low levels in areas of lowest pollution to higher levels in the areas of

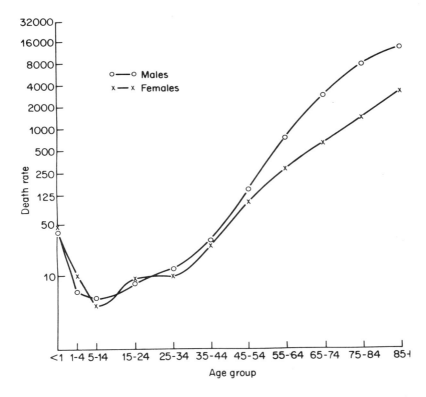

Fig. 6.2   Bronchitis (chronic and unspecified). Emphysema and asthma. Death rates per million living by age and sex. (Data from OPCS.)

Table 6.3   Standardized mortality ratios for chronic bronchitis and emphysema (ICCD nos 490—492) by standard regions in England and Wales, 1978. (Derived from *Mortality Statistics*, Area: (DHS No. 5), Table 3, OPCS.)

Region	Standardized mortality ratio	
	Males	Females
North	125	124
Yorkshire and Humberside	117	118
East Midlands	95	93
East Anglia	75	75
South East	88	94
Greater London (included in South East)	97	116
South West	70	63
West Midlands	113	97
North West	122	128

highest pollution, with a three-fold difference between the two extremes. At the medical examinations carried out at fifteen years, physical signs of respiratory tract infection, or its after-effects, were found most often in children from high pollution areas, suggesting that the effects were long lasting.

Fairbairn and Reid (1958) demonstrated that postmen living in areas similar to those which Howe has shown to have high SMRs from bronchitis had increased sickness rates. Their map based on sickness rates in postmen is strikingly similar to Howe's map of bronchitis mortality. In recent studies by OPCS based upon the collection of occupational mortality data in association with the 1971 census, clear evidence emerged that exposure to atmospheric pollution was associated with increased mortality from the group of diseases categorized as 'bronchitis, emphysema and asthma'. Pollution by dust seemed more important than pollution by fumes (OPCS, 1978).

As the quality of the air in our towns is improved by the increasing implementation of the Clean Air Act 1956 and subsequent associated legislation, the cigarette is taking over as the major identifiable environmental factor in relation to chronic bronchitis. The association with the smoking of cigarettes has been noted by many workers, and not only in the United Kingdom. In the extensive study by Hammond and Horn carried out in the U.S.A. an excess of deaths from respiratory diseases, including bronchitis, was noted in smokers. Doll and Hill in Britain, and Dorn in the U.S.A. showed that death rates from bronchitis and emphysema are related to the numbers of cigarettes smoked (Royal College of Physicians (1971), *Smoking and Health Now*, p. 72). A study reported by Palmer (1954) showed that the prevalence of bronchitis was higher amongst the 310 smokers in a group of 422 males than it was in the non-smokers; the difference was statistically significant. Cigarette smokers tend to cough more and produce more sputum than non-smokers almost as soon as they take up the habit, and tend to have more chest illnesses.

Objective assessments of lung function may be made by measuring the peak expiratory flow achievable by an individual and the vital capacity of the lungs as measured by the maximum volume of air which can be expired. Such measurements demonstrate that the function of the lungs is impaired in cigarette smokers, and this impairment is demonstrable at quite an early stage. In an American study, Janet Seeley and co-workers investigated 365 teenagers ranging in age from 15 to 19. Fifty per cent of the boys and 37% of the girls were regular smokers. Measuring maximum expiratory flow rates and vital capacity they demonstrated that those with five years smoking experience had reduced flow rates at mid-vital capacity and lower lung volumes. They came to the conclusion that their findings probably indicated small airway obstruction in the smokers. Very similar findings were made in studies in the United Kingdom based in Staveley, Derbyshire, where surveys of chronic respiratory disease were conducted in 1957 and in 1966 in representative samples of the male populations. Of the 756 men originally examined in 1957, 594 (78.6%) were seen again in 1966 as part of the new 1966 sample of 992 men. The assessments included records of respiratory symptoms, chest illnesses and smoking habits, and the forced expiratory volume and forced vital capacity were measured. Cough, sputum, wheezing, breathlessness and the occurrence of chest illnesses were all greater in the smokers than in the non-smokers, and their forced expiratory volumes were reduced.

According to the Royal College of Physicians 1977 Report, *Smoking or Health*, a non-smoker who finds himself in a small enclosed space such as a railway compartment, car or small office, in company with several heavy smokers, may in one hour inhale as much smoke as an average smoker inhales from one cigarette. Such 'passive' smoking is theoretically capable of causing some damage to health, since it is just another way of inhaling polluted air. There is some evidence from studies of children who are passive smokers that they suffer as a result. As part of a general follow-up study of newborn infants and their families living in Harrow, northwest London, the incidence of bronchitis and pneumonia was studied in 2205 infants over the first year of life. The occurrence of these conditions was directly associated with the smoking habits of their parents. Thus the children of non-smoking parents had the lowest incidence and where both parents smoked the incidence was highest. Furthermore, the risk of the baby having chest infections was intermediate where only one parent smoked. (Colley *et al.*, 1973). In a similar study (Harlop and Davies, 1974), babies whose mothers smoked were found to be at greater risk of admission to hospital for the treatment of bronchitis or pneumonia, especially during the winter. Colley has also demonstrated that school age children of smokers are at greater risk of respiratory tract infection.

6.4 Allergic lung diseases

Animal and vegetable dusts, including mould spores and pollen grains, may be small enough to remain airborne for considerable periods of time and to penetrate the defences of the respiratory tract. Pollen grains trapped in the nasal passages causing local sensitization and irritation lead to the typical clinical picture of hay fever, but these and other allergens penetrating into the bronchioles may cause symptoms of partial airway obstruction due to contraction of the muscles controlling the diameter of the bronchioles. This again may lead to local obstruction and tissue damage predisposing to secondary infection. Wheezing accompanied by difficulty in emptying the lungs because of bronchospasm, and resultant 'blown up' lungs is the syndrome of asthma. About half of all cases of asthma can be attributed to immunological hypersensitivity reactions to allergens in the environment which lead to the release of chemical mediators of inflammation and bronchospasm. The allergens may be plant pollens, fungal spores, or house dust. In the latter an important part is played by a tiny but ubiquitous mite, *Dermatophagoides pteronyssinus* (Fig. 6.3), which, amongst other habitats, favours mattresses. It also seems to occur with greater frequency and in greater concentrations in damp houses, which might account in part for the popular association of dampness with respiratory tract infections. Animal danders and feathers are also potential allergens, and these, as well as those others mentioned above, may also be responsible for hay fever in susceptible individuals.

A similar type of condition caused by abnormal immunological response is known as extrinsic allergic alveolitis. Here the changes affect the alveolar tissues of the lungs rather than the bronchi and bronchioles, leading to recurrent bouts of respiratory discomfort and possibly some more generalized symptoms such as fever and, if repeated frequently, to a progressive disability caused by summating damage to the lung tissues.

'Farmers lung' was so named after it had been first described in a group of farmers who suffered from acute respiratory symptoms whenever they were exposed to mouldy hay. The symptoms do not appear until several hours after the

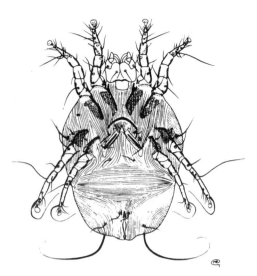

Fig. 6.3 *Dermatophagoides pteronyssinus*, the house dust mite. (After Fain, 1966. Reproduced by permission of the Trustees of the British Museum, from Smith, Kenneth, G.V. (Ed.) (1973). *Insects and other Arthropods of Medical Importance*.)

exposure, but there then follows a bout of respiratory discomfort, cough, and fever, which may persist for several days. The antigen causing the condition is produced by certain thermophilic actinomycetes which grow well in warm fermenting hay. A similar condition, bagassosis, occurs in workers who handle cane fibre. This is a by-product of sugar cane refining, and often becomes wet and mouldy because it is stored out of doors. Here also, the allergen appears to be derived from a thermophilic actinomycete. It seems likely that the disturbance of the wet hay or bagasse produces a local aerosol containing the actinomycetes which is then inhaled by the victim.

'Pigeon fanciers lung' is yet another variety of allergic alveolitis, caused in this case by dust derived from pigeons. 'Humidifier fever' (see p. 40) associated with the use of air conditioning systems which incorporate water sprays to humidify the air pumped around the system is another example, caused by the dispersal of water dwelling organisms into the circulating air.

6.5   The pneumoconioses

Pneumoconiosis is a general term describing disease of the lungs caused by various particles which are inhaled and accumulate in bronchioles and alveoli whence they cannot be expelled, since they are below the level at which the 'respiratory escalator' functions. Many inhaled dusts accumulate in the lungs without stimulating any local reaction, and so do not lead to recognizable or progressive disease. The lungs of town dwellers commonly contain accumulations of dark material, possibly derived from soot and grime in the atmosphere. Workers may be exposed to dust clouds, particles from which may enter their lungs but lead to no lasting disease, although they may lead to opacities visible in X-ray pictures of their chests, a condition of 'benign pneumoconiosis'. Such relatively benign dusts include those containing calcium based materials (e.g. limestone, cement, gypsum and marble) and certain metals or their oxides (e.g. iron, tin, or antimony). The extent of this variety of pneumoconiosis is determined only by the frequency, intensity and duration of exposure of the worker. Dust control or other means of preventing exposure will prevent further deterioration, although once implanted the dust remains and the lesions can never improve. However, other forms of pneumoconiosis may not be limited by cessation of exposure, but may develop a more progressive character, owing to local tissue reactions which are provoked by the presence of the foreign material.

Silicosis   Silica exists in nature in many forms, but it is mainly free silica which leads to damage in lung tissues. Minerals such as quartz, coesite, cristobile and tridymite are important sources of free silica and are therefore potentially dangerous. Exposure to free silica is an occupational hazard in a number of occupations (Table 6.4). Lung tissues react to the presence of silica by forming localized nodules

Table 6.4   Occupations in which exposure to silica dust is a potential hazard.

Quarrying	Sandstone	Slate
	Granite	
Mining	Gold	Coal
	Tin	Graphite
	Iron ore	Slate
Processes	Tile making	Millstone dressing
	Glass manufacture	Sandblasting
	Flint crushing	Metal grinding
	Silica milling	Abrasive soap manufacture
	Silica brick manufacture	Iron and steel smelting
	and furnace lining	

of tissues around the particles. The nodules tend to enlarge and run together, so blotting out areas of lung tissue and impairing the respiratory function of the lungs. In time the nodules become infiltrated and distorted by scar tissue (fibrosis). Silicosis takes many years to develop to the stage where obvious disability is caused; cessation of exposure at a relatively early stage of development will prevent further deterioration, but by the time the first recognizable symptoms of disease appear the condition will already be well advanced, will probably progress further, and the victim is virtually certain to end his or her life as a respiratory cripple. There is also a strong tendency for tuberculosis of the lungs to develop as a complication. Silicosis is frequently complicated by chronic bronchitis, especially if the affected person is also a cigarette smoker. Thus adequate protection at work to reduce the risk of inhaling silica laden dust to the absolute minimum is essential.

Asbestosis   Asbestos is a mineral consisting of a variety of types. It is an extremely useful material for purposes of insulation, and for use in special building materials such as roofing panels, cements, fire proof tiles and paints, brake linings, acid resistant clothing, fire fighting suits, fireproof curtains in theatres, and the like. Small wonder that it is very widely used, and that a substitute would be difficult to find.

However, accumulation of significant quantities of asbestos fibres in the lungs leads to a local tissue reaction which consists mainly of a diffuse fibrosis and thickening of the walls of the alveoli. Under the microscope the fibres may be easily seen lying in the thickened walls of affected alveoli. The fibrotic process particularly affects the lower parts of the lungs. Asbestosis may sometimes be complicated by the occurrence of superadded lung cancer. Doll (1955) showed that the risk of lung cancer developing in asbestos workers who had been exposed for more than 20 years was ten times that of the general population, and this finding was confirmed by an American study published some nine years later (Selikoff *et al.*, 1964). Again, cigarette smoking appears to enhance the risk, as if asbestosis and cigarette smoke act synergistically. It should also be remembered that, quite apart from the massive industrial type of exposure which leads to asbestosis, some individuals may develop the cancerous condition of mesothelioma following exposure to quite small quantities of asbestos dust (see Chap. 4). Asbestos is thus increasingly regarded as a potentially dangerous material, to be handled carefully, with full protection against the generation of dust, and the inhalation and indeed ingestion of its fibres.

Coal workers pneumoconiosis   The dust of coal mines produces fibrosis of lung tissue if exposure goes on over a long period of time. The presence of silicates in the rock from which the coal is mined may play its part but may not be essential, and when examined in detail, the lesions of coal workers pneumoconiosis are distinguishable from those of silicosis. The net result is, however, similar, with localized, heavily pigmented foci of dust accumulation and tissue reaction in or near the bronchioles, often associated with distortion of nearby alveolar structure. The dust is actually held within large phagocytic cells (macrophages) which lie within areas of fibre formation, and it is probably the gradual shortening of these fibres as they mature which distorts the local alveoli. With continuing exposure to coal dust the deposition of fibrous tissue increases and may go on to obliterate whole areas of lung tissue. This slowly undermines the respiratory efficiency of the lungs and renders them prone to intercurrent infection. The end result may be severe respiratory disability.

Beryliosis   A rare but more recently recognized form of pneumoconiosis is that attributable to exposure to the metal beryllium, its oxide, or other compounds of the metal. There is an acute form of beryllium intoxication which arises within some 72 hours of exposure to its fumes, and which itself may be very serious, but the pneumoconiotic process appears many years after exposure, possibly up to 17 years later. Local lesions and areas of infiltration by cells and fibrous tissue appear in the lungs. The victim develops a chronic cough and a progressive tendency to be short of breath. The condition is progressive once it has commenced, even in the absence of further exposure. The underlying pathology of the condition is ill understood.

Beryllium is used as the source of incandescence in flourescent lights, and exposure usually occurs in the metal extraction and smelting industry, although cases have occurred in association with the making of alloys containing beryllium, and even amongst people living close to beryllium extraction plants.

7
Accidents

In England and Wales, about 20 000 people die as a result of violence every year. Three quarters of these deaths are the result of an accident. Hundreds of thousands suffer accidental injury of greater or lesser severity, and a proportion of these end up with permanent disability. The pattern has changed very little from year to year since the beginning of the century (Table 7.1). During the first five years of the 1970s, the situation remained much the same; there were on average 21 763 deaths per annum from violence of which 16 292 (64.9%) were due to accidents.

Table 7.1 Average of deaths from violence and accidents, in decades, 1900—70 in England and Wales (OPCS data).

Decade	Deaths from violence (average)	Deaths from accident (average)	Per cent accidents
1901—10	19 549	15 762	80.6
1911—20	21 107	15 976	75.7
1921—30	19 167	14 489	75.6
1931—40	25 731	17 461	67.9
1941—50	27 006	15 898	58.9
1951—60	21 260	15 800	74.3
1961—70	23 271	17 350	73.1

In 1979, there were 21 753 deaths from violence, of which 15 454 (71%) were accidental (Table 7.2). Numerically most important were motor vehicle traffic accidents, almost as numerous were accidental deaths attributable to falls. These two categories alone accounted for 68% of the accidental deaths during the year; taken singly, other causes were very much less significant, although in sum they accounted for an additional 5000 deaths (Table 7.3).

Table 7.2 Deaths from violence in England and Wales in 1979 (OPCS data).

	Males	Females	Persons	Per cent
Accidents	8 989	6 465	15 454	71.0
Suicide	2 564	1 631	4 195	19.2
Homicide	280	243	523	2.4
Legal intervention	2	0	2	—
Injury, cause uncertain	860	704	1 564	7.2
War (including late effects)	15	0	15	0.1
All violence	12 710	9 043	21 753	100.0

Table 7.3   Main categories of accidental deaths in England and Wales in 1979 (OPCS data).

	Males	Females	Persons	Per cent
Motor vehicle traffic				
(including pedal cyclists)	4 162	1 682	5 844	37.8
Falls	1 616	3 046	4 662	30.2
Submersion or suffocation	695	395	1 090	7.1
Effects of fire or flames	340	427	767	5.0
Poisoning	397	356	753	4.9
Effects of natural or				
environmental factors	229	254	483	3.1
All other causes	1 550	305	1 855	12.0
All accidents	8 989	6 465	15 454	100.0

Table 7.4 summarizes the two most important causes of death in various sex and age groups, and illustrates the importance of 'accidents, poisonings and violence' as the principal group of causes in males between the ages of one and 34 years. Similarly in females, violence, which as we have seen is predominatly accidental in nature, is the prime cause of death between the ages of one and 24, and second only to cancer between the ages of 25 and 34. A more detailed examination of the age and sex incidence of accidental death reveals that more males than females die from this cause and that the death rates tend to be higher in early adulthood and at the upper end of the age scale, especially the latter (Table 7.5).

The importance of accidents as a cause of death and disability in the young is

Table 7.4   The two principal causes of mortality in each age and sex group in England and Wales.

Age group	Males		Females	
	First	Second	First	Second
1—4	Accidents Poisoning Violence	Respiratory diseases	Accidents Poisoning Violence	Respiratory diseases
5—24	Accidents Poisoning Violence	Cancer	Accidents Poisoning Violence	Cancer
25—34	Accidents Poisoning Violence	Cancer	Cancer	Accidents Poisoning Violence
35—54	Circulatory diseases	Cancer	Cancer	Circulatory diseases
55—74	Circulatory diseases	Cancer	Circulatory diseases	Cancer
75 and over	Circulatory diseases	Respiratory diseases	Circulatory diseases	Respiratory diseases

Table 7.5 Death rates per million by age and sex (M = male, F = female) from certain types of accidents in England and Wales in 1979 (OPCS data).

		<1	1–4	5–14	15–24	25–34	35–44	45–54	55–64	65–74	75–84	85–
Transport accidents	M	28	48	78	404	183	135	131	175	191	348	428
	F	20	38	36	79	40	34	45	65	127	207	193
Motor vehicle traffic accidents	M	28	48	72	385	165	116	115	157	179	325	395
	F	20	37	33	76	37	32	43	62	126	204	193
Accidental poisoning	M	3	3	2	21	24	20	16	18	19	34	67
	F	–	4	2	8	12	16	26	18	22	28	16
Accidental falls	M	6	10	5	12	22	31	40	77	150	608	2485
	F	3	4	2	4	4	9	25	42	145	802	3252
Accidents with fire and flames	M	6	22	6	6	6	8	9	19	32	73	235
	F	20	15	5	5	5	7	8	14	27	97	143
Natural and environmental factors	M	32	2	0	2	3	4	8	13	19	81	243
	F	30	–	0	–	1	1	3	10	18	58	182
Drowning and submersion	M	9	23	15	14	10	8	5	7	10	15	50
	F	10	8	1	1	2	2	4	3	3	11	5
Machinery, cutting and piercing instruments	M	–	1	4	9	9	11	11	10	5	3	–
	F	–	1	1	–	1	0	–	1	–	1	–
All above	M	112	157	182	853	422	333	335	476	605	1487	3903
	F	103	107	80	173	102	101	154	215	468	1408	3984

particularly worth noting. Young people have had less experience of the world, are naturally inquisitive and exploratory, and tend to be more adventurous than their elders. Indeed, they frequently court danger for the sheer thrill of the challenge. Often there is an element of self assertion and competition which may lead to deliberate risk taking. Children are still under the supervision and guardianship of their parents, and are thus protected, but as independence is gained in teens and early twenties, risk taking seems to increase, and the incidence of accidents rises. At the other end of the age scale, increasing impairment of the sensory organs, leading to deteriorating vision or hearing, and to greater instability and reduced motility, lead in their turn to greater proneness to falls. Bones are more fragile because of senile osteomalacia (softening of bone), fractures heal less readily, and prolonged immobilization following upon injury may open the way for respiratory tract infections.

Table 7.6   Social class distribution of accidental death in England and Wales, 1970—72. Standardized mortality ratios for men, aged 15—64 years (OPCS data).

	Social class					
	I	II	IIIN	IIIM	IV	V
Motor vehicle traffic accidents	77	83	89	105	121	174
Accidental falls	49	47	46	103	131	265
Accidental poisoning (drugs etc)	123	100	103	60	109	231
Accidental poisoning (gases)	66	82	81	90	119	184

Table 7.6 gives details of the social class distribution of some types of accident and Fig. 7.1 illustrates the distribution of accidental deaths, poisoning and violence by social class. The gradient of mortality in men, rising from social class II through to social class V is indicative of the importance of social and environmental factors

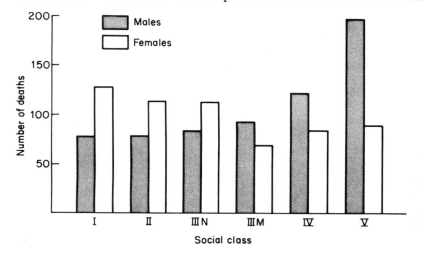

Fig. 7.1   Deaths from accidents, poisoning and violence by social class. Males, SMRs. Females, classified by husband's occupation (SMRs). (Data from OPCS.)

in the causation of accidents. Since the classification is based largely on occupation, hazards encountered at work play their part in the higher rates seen in classes IV and V, along with other factors, such as life in a busy urban environment. Attention to, acceptance of, and compliance with all forms of training and education, aimed at increasing safety consciousness, may also vary across the social spectrum.

Many factors contribute to the occurrence and to the effects of an accident. When thinking about these it is useful to consider three phases related to the occurrence of the accident: the build-up phase; the accident itself; and its aftermath (Fig. 7.2). The accident itself occupies an extremely short period of time, usually

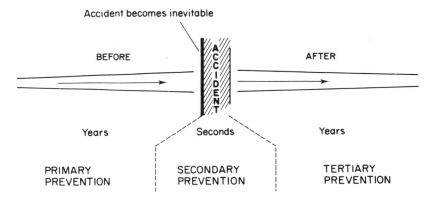

Fig. 7.2   Accident profile.

measured in seconds or fractions of a second, but the phases before and after spread over a very much longer period. The first phase may spread over a number of years preceding the actual accident, associated factors becoming more critical as the moment of the accident approaches. In the final moments several factors may combine coincidentally to precipitate the event; the absence of one or more of these might well have prevented it from occurring at all. However, as the critical combination is reached at a specific point in time the accident can no longer be avoided. This is the moment of inevitability, indicated on the diagram. The accident then occurs over a very brief period of time, and is immediately followed by the third phase which again may last for a very long period, possibly running into many years.

Primary prevention is possible only up to the moment of inevitability; from there on secondary prevention will be important, aimed at reducing the bad effects of the accident to the minimum possible, for example protection against the effects of an impact by padding or protective clothing, or assisting individuals to stay afloat in a water based accident by ensuring that they are equipped with efficient life jackets. Once the accident has occurred, rescue, treatment and rehabilitation come into play as tertiary preventive measures. The objective now must be to prevent further deterioration of those injured, to reduce the risk of complications ensuing, and to obtain the maximum degree of recovery possible. The relevant activities will be most intense immediately after the occurrence of the accident, but may persist for a long time afterwards and, where serious disability has resulted, may never entirely cease.

7.1   Motor vehicle traffic accidents

In 1979 motor vehicle accidents claimed nearly six thousand lives, representing 38% of all accidental deaths (see Table 7.3). As the number of vehicles on the roads has increased over the years, so the relative importance of motor accidents has increased (Table 7.7). This may not be surprising, but must none-the-less be disappointing, since it indicates a continuing failure of adaptation to an important change in the environment. Figure 7.3 demonstrates the age and sex distribution of motor vehicle accident deaths. It is apparent that two peaks of risk occur, in the 15 to 24 age group and in the elderly aged 75 and over. At all ages, males are at greater risk than females. The social class distribution of mortality is similar to that of all violence, with the main risk of death falling in social classes IV and V (Fig. 7.4).

About 33% of all the fatalities on the road are pedestrians, and of these 20% are children. Five per cent of road fatalities are pedal cyclists, 20% are motor cyclists.

Table 7.7   Percentage of accidental deaths due to road transport accidents in England and Wales, by decade, 1900–70. (OPCS data.)

Decade	All accidents	Road transport accidents	Percentage road transport accidents
1901–1910	15 762	2 475	15.7
1911–1920	15 976	3 537	22.1
1921–1930	14 481	4 430	30.6
1931–1940	17 461	6 531	37.4
1951–1960	15 800	5 288	33.5
1961–1970	17 350	6 946	40.0

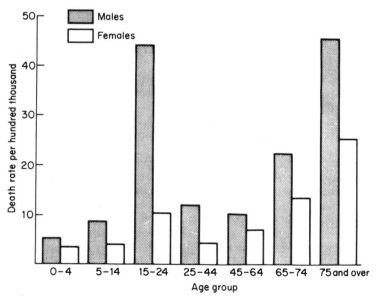

Fig. 7.3   Histogram of death rates from road traffic accidents in England and and Wales within specific age and sex groups, 1978. (Data from OPCS.)

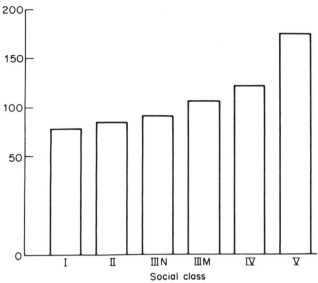

Fig. 7.4 Mortality from motor vehicle traffic accidents in England and Wales; males, aged 15–64, by social class (SMRs). (From OPCS, 1978.)

The proportion of motor cyclists has shown an increase in recent years as the number of travellers turning to this mode of transport has increased, no doubt for economic reasons. Over all the categories of road accidents, children account for some 10% of fatalities.

Quite apart from those actually killed, road traffic accidents exact a heavy toll of injuries. In all, over 300 000 persons are injured in a year, 80 000 (27%) seriously. A residuum of disabilities ranging from amputated limbs to severe brain damage and mental handicap persists. Pedestrians account for 25% of those seriously injured, and motor cyclists for another 25%. Children account for about 14% of serious injuries. This shows a clear failure of the human race to adapt to and live safely with an environmental factor of its own making, because the time scale in which it has occurred is much too short. Rather, they have tended to adapt to the effects; the motor car and the motor cycle seem to have become an accepted way of death. There are no public protests or public marches about the continuing carnage on the roads, where on average sixteen people are killed every day.

In considering the environmental influences at work in the genesis of motor vehicle accidents, it will be helpful to use the accident profile as a skeleton on which to hang the analysis. The factors in each phase may be considered under the headings of the vehicle, the human element, and the road (Table 7.8).

Phase 1.   Before: opportunities for primary prevention

Good vehicle design, which enhances stability and road holding qualities, enables effective control to be maintained while the vehicle is in motion. An effective braking system is clearly important, including special systems such as the anti jack-knifing gear built into some articulated lorries. Good visibility all round is also an important design feature, together with an effective lighting system. Good

Table 7.8   Environmental factors in road traffic accidents.

	Vehicle	Human	Road
BEFORE (Primary prevention)	Design Stability Road holding Power Visibility Brakes Lights Tyres Maintenance Regular service Competent mechanics Training of mechanics	Drivers Adequate training Psychology Attitude Physical fitness Fatigue Emotional stress Alcohol Drugs Pedestrians Training Awareness Physical fitness (age) Fatigue Emotional stress Alcohol Drugs	Design and construction Carriageway Surface Visibility Intersections Corners Traffic control equipment Signs Maintenance
DURING (Secondary prevention)	Design Stability Braking efficiency Steering control Tyres Built-in protection Strong passenger compartment 'Crumple zones' Triplex glass Seat belts Door locks	Reflexes Training Psychology Physical fitness	Weather State of surface Space Presence of 'escape route'
AFTER (Tertiary prevention)	Design Ease of ingress for rescue Fire resistance	Psychology Training (first aid) Medical and rescue services	Communications Space for access to accident

and regular maintenance, particularly of tyres, steering, brakes, and lights, is important to keep the vehicle in a safe condition.

The human element includes the driver of a vehicle, pedal cyclists and pedestrians. Drivers must be adequately trained and well tested for their competence to drive. Apart from the technical ability needed to control a vehicle and negotiate traffic and other hazards encountered when driving, the psychological make up of drivers and their general approach to driving is important. Everyone who drives a car is aware of the competitive element in driving, the temptation to take a pride in a person's driving 'ability' and to denigrate that of others. This dangerous tendency is heightened by the circumstances of driving, possibly in congested conditions, and the inability to communicate effectively with other road users. Misunderstandings about the intentions or motives of other drivers, and misinterpretation of their actions may lead to impatience and petulance.

Closely allied to this aspect of driver psychology is the tendency, perhaps particularly amongst younger persons, to knowingly take risks. The thrill of fear, or the enjoyment of a challenging situation, coupled with the sense of achievement in 'getting away with it' may lead some individuals into dangerous situations. Such risk taking may stem from a desire to prove oneself, and to earn the admiration of others as courageous, intrepid, or daring. This rather immature attitude may be found in some young people, but not exclusively so. It is a potential danger to all drivers, for few have not experienced the desire to be competitive when driving a car, to be a better driver than the next man, which often means to get somewhere more quickly, to 'beat the others to it', and possibly to take unjustifiable risks along the way as a result.

Insufficient attention is paid to the psychology of driving. Perhaps a driver's training should include explicit discussion of these issues, and perhaps part of the assessment of a person's ability to drive should be a psychological assessment to identify those who might become aggressive in difficult situations, or who might be tempted to drive competitively. Such concepts are radical, but may need consideration. There is clear physiological evidence that when a person is driving, changes occur in pulse rate and blood pressure indicating that the adrenaline like effects of the primitive 'fight or flight' reflex are active. They are seen at their most pronounced in racing car drivers just before the start of a race, but are detectable in drivers in ordinary traffic conditions, and become more pronounced as traffic conditions become more difficult.

Any form of psychological distress, or fatigue, may impair concentration and judgement. Another important factor which often affects judgement is alcohol. The euphoria which alcohol usually produces leads to a lessening of the appreciation of potentially dangerous circumstances, and so increases risk taking behaviour. At the same time, judgement of space and speed is impaired, and self confidence is inflated. This is a most dangerous combination, and experience shows that consumption of alcohol is a contributor to a significant proportion of motor vehicle accidents. The Road Safety Act 1967, tightened up the law relating to drinking and driving, and created new offences of driving, attempting to drive, or being in charge of a motor vehicle while the proportion of alcohol in the blood is in excess of 80 mg per 100 ml. The new legislation came into force on October 9th 1967, when the breathalyser test was introduced. The effects of this were interesting (Table 7.9). Up to October 8th there had been a reduction of 1.6% in deaths and 2.1% in non-fatal accidents by comparison with the same period in the previous year. From October 9th to the end of the year fatalities decreased by 25% and injuries by 15.9% over the corresponding period of 1966. Deaths on the road over the Christmas period fell by 35.9% by comparison with Christmas 1966. Since that time, drivers have found weaknesses in the legislation and have also come to realise that there are difficulties in enforcement. Some are therefore prepared to 'take a chance'. The initial effect of the drink and drive laws has largely disappeared. Improved legislation is under consideration, but at the end of the day it is personal behaviour and the personal sense of responsibility which is most important.

Similar conditions apply to pedestrians and pedal cyclists. General physical fitness, and awareness are also important. Impaired hearing, vision, or mobility may render them more vulnerable to traffic accidents. Children must be carefully trained to cope with traffic. Fatigue or preoccupation with other matters can undermine attention, or distract.

Table 7.9 Total occurrence of road traffic accidents in England and Wales by month of occurrence, 1966 and 1967.

Month	1966	1967	Increase (+) Decrease (−)
January	27 031	27 493	+ 462
February	26 268	27 208	+ 940
March	29 831	30 199	+ 368
April	32 568	28 553	−4015
May	35 151	34 085	−1066
June	34 415	30 884	−3531
July	35 671	34 677	− 994
August	33 555	33 737	+ 182
September	31 911	33 560	+1649
October	31 911	22 560	+1649
November	33 374	28 880	−4494
December	37 562	29 707	−7855

Road conditions are most important in the primary prevention of accidents. The carriageway should be designed in such a way as to allow plenty of space and good visibility. The gradual trend away from two way roads to dual carriageways which separate traffic travelling in opposite directions is to be welcomed. Future generations may well consider our present practice of driving at high speeds in opposite directions at the same time to be an incredible form of lunacy. Most notorious of all is the three lane two way carriageway where the centre lane is intended for overtaking in either direction. This proved to be a death trap for many unwary or unduly adventurous motorists. Good corner and road junction design, allowing good visibility and complementing the road holding qualities of vehicles, the qualities of the road surface, particularly its coefficient of friction, and its drainage characteristics, are all design factors very relevant to accident prevention. Apart from good design, good maintenance of roads is important, keeping the surface in good order and ensuring that warning signs and lighting remain effective.

Phase 2.   During: Secondary prevention

Once the accident becomes inevitable, factors which will reduce the effects upon those involved become operative. In terms of the design of the vehicle, a stronger passenger compartment, protected by 'crumple zones' fore and aft to absorb the energy of the impact as much as possible, is an important factor. Most modern vehicles have this kind of protection built into them. Strong door locks will resist pressures tending to burst the doors open, effective seat belts will stop those inside from being thrown about in or, even worse, out of the vehicle, and steering columns should be designed to give way before they cause serious damage to the chest of the driver. Good braking and steering qualities assist the driver to make the maximum possible reduction in speed before impact and to possibly avoid a head-on collision. The interior of the vehicle can be padded, especially over angles and projections, to further reduce the risk of injury, and the petrol tank and connections to carburettor and engine should be designed to be flexible yet strong, in order to keep to a minimum any risk of petrol leakage and resultant fire.

Drivers and passengers should be encouraged to wear protective devices such as seat belts. A considerable amount of evidence has been amassed, both experimentally and as a result of accident investigations, showing that the risk of injury or death, whilst not eliminated, is considerably reduced if seats belts are worn. Very serious injuries can be caused by impact with the interior of the vehicle, or by being thrown out, possibly through the windscreen. Following failure of attempts to induce their use voluntarily, legislation passed in 1981 made them compulsory (see page 116).

Perhaps part of driver training should include instruction on how to act in the event of an imminent accident. At present there seem to be no rules. For example, if vehicle A is being overtaken by vehicle B which is suddenly in danger of head-on collision with a third approaching vehicle, C, should A slow down? However, this might prevent B from falling behind in order to avoid collision with C. Should A accelerate? But perhaps B decides to accelerate too, intending to try to cut in front of A. Should there be some consideration of these issues by driving instructors? It is noteworthy that the pilots of aircraft are trained to handle emergencies efficiently, and that fewer people are killed flying than driving on the roads.

The road surface also plays its part in determining the outcome of the crash, and those aspects of design and maintenance which are important in primary prevention are clearly of equal importance in the second phase of the accident profile.

Phase 3.   Afterwards: Tertiary prevention

When all has come to rest, the third phase is concerned with preventing any further aggravation of the injuries which have been caused, and with avoiding complications and keeping the costs of the accident as low as possible. Avoidance of secondary accidents may depend heavily upon warning procedures, and these in turn depend upon effective communications. The amount of space and visibility available are also vital at this time. The major multiple crashes which have occurred on motorways affected by fog are an extreme example of this kind of problem. Communications and the design and maintenance of the road will also affect the speed with which police and ambulance, and, if necessary, the fire brigade can respond. The availability of adequate resources to these services is also clearly important in allowing them to make effective provision.

Avoidance of further injury to those immediately involved will partly depend upon the first aid training of those persons first on the spot. Perhaps this points to a further requirement of a future driving test — the possession of a certificate of competence in simple first aid. Once rescue has been effected by the accident services, the availability of efficient accident and emergency centres in nearby hospitals, with medical and surgical backup for immediate and longer term care, and with associated services for rehabilitation provide the last link in the chain.

7.2   Accidents in the home

At first sight it is perhaps surprising to discover that the home can be as dangerous a place as the road when it comes to the risk of accidental death. Table 7.10 compares the numbers of deaths which have taken place in the home and on the road over recent years. However, as comparison of Fig. 7.3 and 7.5 shows, the age and sex distribution of deaths from accidents on the road and accidents in the home are very different. On the roads, male mortality predominates; in the home, female mortality is higher. On the roads, the principal impact falls on the 75 and over age group but the 15 to 24 age group comes a very close second, and the death rates at

Table 7.10   Comparison of fatal home and road accidents in England and Wales. 'Home' includes residential accommodation. (From *Social Trends*, 1981, Table 8.17.)

Year	Home	Road
1961	6 882	6 778
1966	7 470	7 546
1971	6 245	7 072
1976	5 619	6 115
1977	5 369	5 943
1978	5 341	6 772

the lower end of the age scale are relatively low. In the home, mortality is slightly elevated at the lower end of the age scale and greatly so at the upper. The importance of falls as a cause of death was mentioned early in this chapter, and it is in the home and in the aged that falls become of major importance (Table 7.11, Fig. 7.6). Falls account for 59% of all accidental deaths in the home, but for 79% of those in persons aged 75 and over (Table 7.12).

Poisoning at home is also relatively important as a hazard; it is an important cause of accidents to children, but otherwise affects mainly persons of working age and women (see Table 7.5). Accidents involving fire are also numerically important. These three groups of causes, falls, poisoning, and fire, account for 77% of male and 85% of female accidental deaths in the home.

As with all kinds of accidents, the fatalities are only the tip of the iceberg; there are a vast number of non-fatal accidents requiring treatment every year. Hospital in-patient statistics demonstrate that over a hundred thousand people receive in-patient treatment each year in England and Wales, and the Royal Society for the Prevention of Accidents estimate that, in the whole of Great Britain 700 000 persons are treated as hospital outpatients, and a further 500 000 are treated by their family doctors following accidents at home.

An analysis of the potential factors relating to home accidents reveals considerable complexity. The most dangerous places in the home are stairways and the kitchen. A review of the factors in depth requires specific attention to these locations and possibly even to specific areas within them. Table 7.13 examines factors in a general way, utilizing the accident profile as a framework. In this instance the factors in each part of the profile relate to the premises and to the victim. As far as the home itself is concerned, good design suited to the capacities of the occupants is a major requirement, but equally important is the need to maintain the premises and contents in good repair. Stairways should be straight and well lit, with even risers and treads and good non-slip floor surfaces. Glass doors may be decorative and useful for improving the light of stairwells, but they present a major hazard if they are located, for instance, at the bottom of a flight of stairs. Annealed or tempered glass must be used in glass doors.

Windows should open easily, yet have secure fastenings, and should not be so placed that it would be easy to fall out of them. There should be adequate space where children can play in safety and preferably under observation; whether there are young or old in a family it is an advantage to have a toilet downstairs. Gas and electrical mains must be kept in good repair. Numerous other factors need to be kept in mind when considering specific rooms in a house (Table 7.13).

Much also depends upon the condition of the potential accident victim. The very

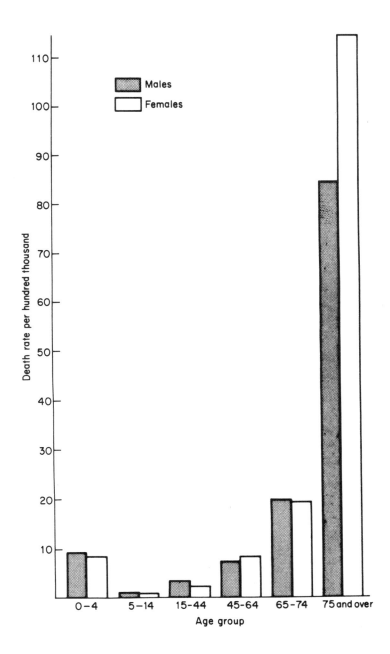

Fig. 7.5 Accidental deaths in the home in England and Wales by age and sex, 1978. (Data from OPCS.)

Table 7.11　Main causes of accidental death in the home in England and Wales, 1978 (OPCS data).

Cause	Number of deaths	
	Males	Females
Accidental poisoning	293	343
Falls	1006	2131
Accidents with fire	267	337
Drowning	40	57
Asphyxiation	194	207
Scald, corrosive burn	15	33
Electrocution	24	7
Other accidents	181	190
All accidents	2028	3313

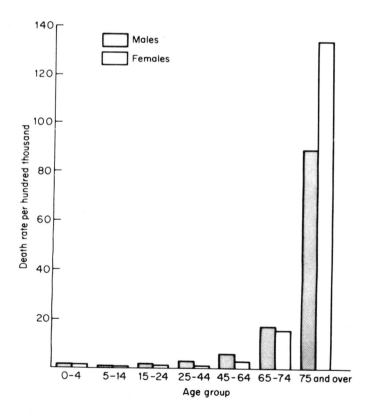

Fig. 7.6　Death rates from falls in England and Wales within specific age and sex groups, 1978. (Data from OPCS.)

Table 7.12 Comparison of death rates of road traffic accidents, falls, and all home accidents by age and sex groups, England and Wales, 1978. Death rates per 100 000 home population. (OPCS data.)

Age group	Population (1000s)	Road traffic accidents		Falls		Home accidents	
		Deaths	Rate	Deaths	Rate	Deaths	Rate
Males							
0– 4	1519.4	78	5.1	13	0.9	139	9.2
5–14	3962.1	325	8.2	21	0.5	40	1.0
15–24	3733.0	1644	44.0	47	1.3 }	354	3.5
25–44	6383.0	764	12.0	151	2.4 }		
45–64	5486.1	565	10.3	316	5.8	392	7.2
65–74	1979.9	444	22.4	325	16.4	386	19.5
75 and over	850.1	386	45.4	752	88.5	717	84.3
Females							
0– 4	1437.2	55	3.8	17	1.2	122	8.5
5–14	3755.6	150	4.0	6	0.1	28	0.8
15–24	3565.7	367	10.3	10	0.3	224	2.3
25–44	6259.3	276	4.4	35	0.6		
45–64	5774.8	404	7.0	140	2.4	365	6.3
65–74	2588.8	353	13.6	385	14.9	490	18.9
75 and over	1822.3	458	25.1	2429	133.3	2084	112.4

old or the very young may be relatively unstable on their feet and thus more prone to falls. In the elderly there are additional potential problems. Impaired vision or impaired hearing interfere with awareness of surroundings and appreciation of danger, as does an impaired sense of smell where gas or smoke could be warnings of impending danger. Appreciation of possible sources of risk can go a long way towards helping to avoid them. Education and training which includes advice and instruction in such matters can be valuable in promoting home safety, always provided, of course, that the recipient of such advice takes due notice of it.

Once a home accident reaches the point of inevitability, then any design features which will ameliorate the effects become important. For instance, if a fall occurs, any features which will serve to reduce the height of the fall, or to cushion the victim will help, whereas sharp edges or angles of fittings or furniture will possibly make injuries worse. If fire breaks out, a small fire extinguisher ready to hand may prove to be worth its weight in gold. Physical fitness will play its part in helping a person to withstand the immediate effects of the accident.

There is little that the victim can do or contribute after an accident has occurred, but it is important that adequate means of communication is available so that help can be summoned.

7.3   Accidents at work

Fewer accidents occur at work than on the road or at home. Table 7.14 lists the industries within which 438 fatal and 251 640 non-fatal industrial accidents occurred in 1979. Very considerable attention has been paid to the prevention of accidents in the work place, culminating in recent years in the Health and Safety at Work *etc.* Act 1974, which is still in the course of implementation. There has, however,

Table 7.13   Environmental factors relating to home accidents.

	The house	The occupants
BEFORE (Primary)	**Design and maintenance** *General* Stairways, handrails, lighting, space Floor surfaces Glass doors, windows and other fittings Mode of opening of windows, accessibility, fastenings Visible play space for children Ground floor toilet accommodation Fuel supplies — electric wiring, gas mains Fire extinguishers, fire doors, fire and smoke warning devices	Age, sex Physical fitness — vision — hearing — sense of smell Mobility — walking aids — wheel chair Mental state Emotional state Fatigue Awareness
	Kitchen Cooking appliances Layout of working surfaces Space, light Storage facilities, site and accessibility Floor surfaces	Attitudes and habits Education } Compliance Training }
	Bathroom Space Handrails Heating arrangements Water temperature Non-slip bath mats Ventilation — especially with gas 'geysers'	
	Living rooms Furnishings, floor coverings Heating appliances Lighting	
DURING (Secondary prevention)	**Design** Hand rails Short flights of stairs Soft furnishings, absence of sharp edges and corners Non-slip surfaces Available fire extinguishers Warning devices in working order	Footwear and clothing Shoes or slippers in good condition with non-slip surfaces Clothing not easily flammable Physical fitness and agility (recovery from falls) 'Presence of mind' Knowledge of use of safety equipment Training
AFTER (Tertiary prevention)	Non-isolation, visible to passers-by Communications — signals, telephone, warning/alarm bells First aid equipment	Knowledge of first aid Availability of assistance Use of medical services (Availability of medical services)

Table 7.14 Industrial accidents in England and Wales, 1979 (from *Social Trends*, 1981, Table 8.23).

Industry	Total accidents	Number of fatal accidents
Manufacturing	168 374	167
Construction	31 804	138
Railways	5 121	39
Coalmining	40 897	46
Quarrying	1 822	12
Agriculture	4 060	36
Totals	252 078	438

been very little reduction in the overall incidence of accidents at work during recent years, and this must be a cause for disappointment. There have been significant improvements in the coal mining and quarrying industries, in each of which the total number of accidents has decreased by a third since 1971.

7.4 Leisure activities and accidents

Accidents also occur, of course, during recreational or leisure activities. In these circumstances there is frequently deliberate risk taking; the challenge is part of the enjoyment of the activity. The attitude to prevention in such circumstances is clearly modified, since a higher element of risk would be acceptable than in everyday activities of a similar nature. Primary prevention thus becomes less important, but secondary prevention assumes very great importance and the provision of very good rescue and first aid services is also essential.

7.5 The human factor in accidents

Study of the relationships and distribution of accidents and their outcomes demonstrates clearly that their occurrence is strongly dictated by environmental factors. Furthermore the environment which predisposes to an accident is frequently almost entirely man-made. In this sense, accidents are a very explicit expression of man's failure to adapt to environmental changes which he himself has initiated (see p. 4). For instance, the introduction of fast moving traffic during the past eighty years or so, with steadily increasing speeds of travel, represents a change which has taken place with extreme rapidity by comparison with the time scale of evolution. Similarly, the appearance and growth of the factory environment, and industrial urbanization has been an abrupt change in human environmental experience. There have been inevitable risks to be taken whilst experimenting with and developing new technology, which has sometimes meant that experimenters have had to venture into unknown situations and learn by experience. Adaptation can only come from adequate study of the influences and actions which result in injury or death, and from the ability to learn from experience. Lessons learnt can be passed on through education and training and by the implementation of improved design. This may be fine in theory, but there seem to be considerable problems in putting it into practice, for, as has been demonstrated, there has been little in the way of significant improvement in the toll of death and injury caused by accidents over the years.

Education may fail for several reasons. In the first instance, we might ask whether enough education is undertaken into accident prevention. Training should start with the young, the curricula of infant and primary schools should be partly geared towards training for life in a potentially dangerous environment. Parents also have a responsibility to teach their children about common dangers; some are better at this than others. Training for specific jobs or skills should contain an element of safety instruction, including discussion of the kind of behaviour which leads to accidents. Also of great importance is the ability and attitude of the recipient of the education or training. Interest, ability to absorb the information, and to remember it, may vary from individual to individual. Last, and by no means least, those given information must be prepared to accept and comply with it. If they are unconvinced or sceptical, or simply cannot be bothered to take the recommended course of action, then the attempt at accident prevention from this direction may fail.

It was necessary to legally enforce the protection of motor cyclists by the use of crash helmets, and subsequently legislation requiring the wearing of seat belts by the front seat passengers in cars was enacted and was implemented early in 1983. Experience has shown that a large proportion of the motoring public would not take these precautions unless legally required to do so, and there has been active resistance to legislation of this kind, legislation which should not have been necessary in any case in a rational society. This failure in compliance has resulted either from ignorance of the facts relating to the relative safety of wearing or not wearing crash helmets or seat belts, or from forgetfulness or apathy. There is also an element of natural resistance to coercion and the mere fact of legislation may encourage resistance to it, on the basis that it represents an unwarrantable incursion into personal freedom. This begs the question of how far the State is entitled to go when legislating for the welfare of its citizens. Although the problems of crash helmets and seat belts have been specifically mentioned, there are many other examples, such as the use of guards on moving machinery, the use of fire guards to protect young children from open fires, the use of flame proof clothing, or the use of correctly rated fuses in electrical appliances.

Perhaps a great deal more investigation is needed into the psychology of motivation, and into understanding the possibly subconsciously protective 'it won't happen to me' syndrome. We all tend to believe that accidents only happen to other people — until our own turn comes.

Part III Assessing the Hazards

8
Clean air, food and water

The natural environment of earth constitutes a closed system in which basic components are constantly recycled. The energy source for the recycling is the sun. Examples of such natural cycles are those related to carbon, nitrogen, oxygen and water, all of which are highly relevant to the maintenance of an environment conducive to life. The whole system is in a state of dynamic equilibrium and is thus subject to change if disturbing influences are superimposed. 'Pollution' is not easily defined, but, in one sense, can be taken as the presence of abnormal quantities of a material due to disturbance of the natural state of equilibrium. Such a disturbance might well be generated by man's activities, since, with his increasing knowledge and power to manipulate matter and energy, he is able to exert substantial influences upon his own environment.

In the late twentieth century, serious suggestions are being made that human activities may start to upset the fundamental ecological balance of this planet. A typical debate of this nature concerns the so-called 'Greenhouse Effect', based on the hypothesis that increasing concentrations of carbon dioxide from the combustion of fossil fuels will alter the balance of recycling maintained by plant photosynthesis and ocean absorption, leading to atmospheric levels 20 to 25% above the present average of about 300 p.p.m. by the end of the century. It is suggested that one consequence of such an increase could be a raising of the global temperature because of increased atmospheric absorption of solar energy re-radiated from the earth's surface at longer wavelengths, leading to a catastrophic rise in sea levels caused by melting of the polar ice-caps. The opposing view predicts equally serious results from an eventual lowering of the earth's temperature through the reflection of the sun's heat by smoke and particulate matter in the air. In this chapter, some of the consequences of man's activity on elements of his environment which are essential to life are examined.

8.1   Pollution of the atmosphere

The effects of air pollution have been noted for centuries; six hundred years ago legislative control was exercised in Britain over the public nuisance of smoke. When, in the early days of the industrial revolution there was a transition to an urban industrial society from the previous rural and agricultural way of life, the problem became much more serious. The influx of people into towns, accompanied by the development of new industrial processes, greatly increased consumption of fuel and the consequent discharge of increasing volumes of waste products to the atmosphere resulted in local accumulations of smoke, grime and chemical fumes, the effects of which are still visible on some of the older buildings in cities. The effects of this activity on the immediate environment were sometimes little short of devastating, although they were essentially local in nature.

Fortunately the natural world possesses great abilities to disperse pollution through the beneficial influences of wind and weather and to mitigate its effects through natural absorption and recirculation processes which together have prevented the fulfillment of some of the worst predictions of disaster. Sometimes, however, these systems are overloaded and break down, as many well-documented episodes in the history of air pollution testify.

The useful heat-producing components of fossil fuels are hydrogen and carbon, which form water vapour and carbon dioxide on combustion. If sulphur is present it will be partially retained in the ash, if any, but will otherwise be emitted as sulphur dioxide/trioxide. Any oxygen content may be available to take part in the combustion process.

In modern times problems that may arise from the burning of fuels for heat production are, for the most part, well understood and can be controlled. The essential principles are to provide a sufficient supply of air, mix it intimately with the fuel and ensure that furnace design allows adequate time for the complete combustion reaction to take place before discharging the waste gases. The production of poisonous carbon monoxide is an indicator of starvation of air for combustion and a serious loss of efficiency. Good furnace design takes account of the need to completely consume smokey volatile material distilled from the fuel and to prevent smoke production from the quenching of burning gases by contact with relatively cool surfaces. Incinerators present more difficult problems because of the highly variable nature of the waste used as 'fuel', but these can still be overcome by adherence to the principles mentioned and the provision of afterburners to consume smoke.

Emissions of grit and dust can be controlled by a variety of engineering techniques, ranging from relatively low-efficiency settling and impingement chambers to bag filters, venturi water scrubbers and electrostatic precipitators with potential efficiencies of 99% or more. Efficiencies of arrestment are greatest with grit particles (> 75 μm diameter), decreasing at the lower range of dust sizes ($1-75$ μm diameter). Particles below 1 μm are usually classified as 'fume' and worthwhile collection efficiencies can only be achieved with the more sophisticated methods mentioned. There has been less success in removing sulphur dioxide from the combustion gases. The usual method of dealing with this problem is to limit low-level concentration by the adoption of 'tall chimney' policies, relying upon the inverse relationship which exists between the square of the effective chimney height and the concentration of the pollutant at ground level. This is disposal by dilution.

Sulphur dioxide and particulates, which have been widely studied because of their potential to harm lung tissues, are no doubt very useful indicators of general pollution levels and SO_2 as a cause of acid rainfall has attracted international attention. These pollutants do not, however, necessarily portray the whole picture. Urban and industrial atmospheres may contain other substances to which the respiratory tract is vulnerable, despite its defence mechanisms and the scavenging activities of alveolar macrophages (see page 89). Nitrogen oxides (NO_x), ozone, carbon monoxide, cadmium, hydrocarbons, asbestos and many other airborne substances may prove harmful if they pollute the atmosphere. Carbon monoxide reacts mainly with haemoglobin, so limiting the supply of oxygen to the tissues of the body; it may be particularly hazardous to sufferers from circulatory or respiratory conditions, or from anaemia, although, of course, it is a danger to all if a concentration builds up or persists. Airborne metals, in fume or organic form, may be absorbed through the respiratory tract and cause toxic effects there and elsewhere. Dust particles such as asbestos can penetrate the airways of the lungs and cause local irritation, or worse (Chap. 6).

The potential for distribution of chemical pollution into the environment exists from accidental leaks or spillages, evaporation during storage, transport accidents or escape from the manufacturing process itself. Secondary pollution may occur when materials are used for the formulation of other products or from the evolution of toxic by-products. Mixtures of pollutants may lead to the production of a more (or less) harmful compound or the synergistic effect of multiple pollutants may increase the damage which they do beyond the sum of their individual effects.

The most immediate risk from airborne toxic chemicals faces those who are exposed to them in the course of their work and the practice of occupational medicine is rightly directed towards their protection. The general public, however, contains groups, such as the very young, the elderly and the disabled, who are likely to be much more susceptible than the, presumably, fit worker in industry, although through dilution they may not be exposed to 'industrial' concentrations. They do not have the benefit of personal protective equipment, controlled exposure and medical surveillance properly afforded to the person who comes into contact with hazardous materials at work and are entitled to expect optimum quality in the air which they have no option but to breath 24 hours a day, seven days a week.

Information on the long-term effects of continuous exposure of the public to very low levels of chemicals is far from complete and the temptation exists to make assumptions by interpolating the results of research into the effects of much higher concentrations to which groups of people may be exposed whilst at work. Certain dangers are associated with this. Firstly, workforces are mobile and there are notorious difficulties in monitoring people over a long period when they have moved to other locations and occupations, so that developing ill-effects, latent for many years, may easily escape detection. Secondly, it cannot be assumed that a linear relationship exists between level of exposure and effect. There are undoubtedly many chemicals for which a true 'no-effect' threshold exists, but the characteristics of the exposure-effect exposure relationship may vary considerably. These are discussed in detail by Duffus (1980).

8.1.1 Lead as a pollutant

Lead has claimed special attention as a pollutant, in view of its recognized toxicity and its occurrence in air, food and water from a range of sources (Fig. 8.1). The debate on the alleged sub-clinical effects of lead on the developing central nervous system of young children has not yet been totally resolved. A number of studies have examined the relationship of blood-lead levels with behavioural characteristics and intelligence, as far as these qualities are capable of precise definition and can be isolated from hereditary and social influences, but there remains lack of agreement in expert scientific circles about the precise interpretation of the results.

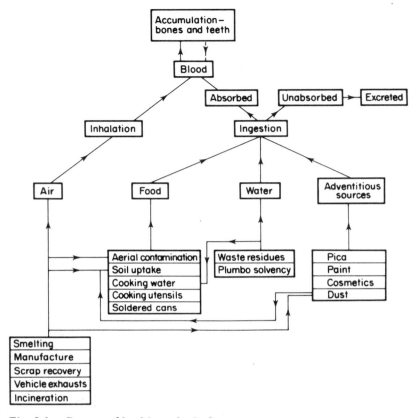

Fig. 8.1   Routes of lead into the body.

There is no dispute about the relative susceptibility of young children to lead, whatever level may ultimately be accepted as safe or otherwise. Their activities tend to expose them to lead in dust and soils and they absorb a much greater proportion of a given level of ingestion (~50%) than do adults (~10%).

It has generally been accepted that blood-lead levels are a reliable indicator of recent bodily absorption, although significant work has been carried out on tooth-lead as an indicator of longer-term exposure. Clinical lead poisoning and encephalopathy occur at blood levels over about 80 μg dl^{-1}, but it is not possible at the present time to predict a threshold for any individual below which the absence of any adverse effect can be guaranteed.

The European Communities have adopted a directive requiring member states to carry out blood-lead surveys on specified groups of the population not occupationally exposed to lead and to take action to trace the source of exposure responsible when the following reference levels are exceeded:

a maximum of 20 μg dl^{-1} for 50% of the group examined
a maximum of 30 μg dl^{-1} for 90% of the group examined
a maximum of 35 μg dl^{-1} for 98% of the group examined
and action in respect of all individuals with a level in excess of 35 μg dl^{-1}

(EEC Directive 77/312/EEC – Lead in Blood Reference Levels)

Government policy in the U.K. requires that where any person, particularly a child, displays a level over 25 μg dl^{-1}, his or her environment must be investigated and steps taken to reduce exposure.

8.1.2   Pollution from motor vehicle emissions

The motor vehicle is a significant contributor to emissions of certain types of pollutant (Table 8.1).

Carbon monoxide	90%
Lead	90%
NO$_x$	25%
Hydrocarbons	30%

Table 8.1   Approximate contribution of motor vehicle exhausts to total mass emissions in the United Kingdom.

In Europe the predominant issue in vehicle emission control has tended to be carbon monoxide, because of concern over conditions in congested and poorly ventilated urban areas where traffic waits with engines idling. In the U.S.A. greater emphasis has been placed on the formation of photochemical smog, with hydrocarbons and oxides of nitrogen being the principal objects of control.

In petrol engines, manipulation of the air/fuel ratio can be used to bring about reductions in either CO, hydrocarbons or NO$_x$, but only at the expense of an increase in the other pollutants, unless advanced engineering techniques are used (Fig. 8.2).

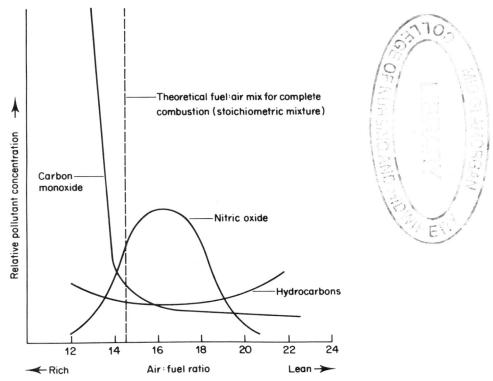

Fig. 8.2   Relative emissions with varying air-fuel ratios (petrol engine). (Courtesy of Dr J.H. Weaving, BL Cars Advanced Technology, from *The Technology of Controlling Exhaust Emissions*, presented at the National Society for Clean Air Spring Workshop, Warwick University, April, 1979.)

The use of a very lean ratio appears to offer an attractive option for the reduction of NO_x at the expense of a relatively modest increase in hydrocarbons. Unfortunately, this leads to serious loss of efficiency, as the rate of heat release from the fuel is slowed. This can be offset by increasing the engine's compression ratio, provided that greater sensitivity in the ignition timing is also achieved, to prevent premature detonation of the fuel/air mixture. More difficult problems are encountered in balancing the richness of the atomized fuel reaching each cylinder, which becomes a critical performance factor in lean-running engines. 'Stratified Charge' engines in which a rich mixture is introduced in the region of the sparking plug with a lean one filling the remainder of the combustion chamber are at present under development and provide an encouraging prospect of cleaner exhaust discharges. A controlling factor will be the costs incurred, either in more sophisticated engineering or reduced efficiency and the public will have to make an educated political choice in this matter.

Cost is also a key consideration in reducing lead emissions from petrol engines. The addition of lead compounds to fuel promotes greater efficiency by permitting the use of higher compression ratios, pre-ignition being controlled by the lead additives. Certainly, the use of lead for this purpose could be curtailed by reverting to reduced efficiency low-compression engines, or by additional refining of crude oil to produce higher-octane motor fuel, at the cost of extra processing losses and a lower overall production of useful products from each barrel of crude. Effective control is also available from the use of exhaust filtration, but carries the penalties of higher initial cost and increased maintenance. Lead causes problems by contaminating lubricating oils and adding to the build-up of deposits within the engine. These effects are partially controlled by scavenging agents which are corrosive not only to the lead deposits, but to the interior of the engine and exhaust system and tend to increase maintenance costs. Such costs would be likely to decrease following the prohibition or drastic reduction of lead addition to petrol and represent an economic benefit to be offset against the costs of such measures. In April 1983, the U.K. Government undertook to discuss with oil producers and the motor industries a timetable for the introduction of unleaded petrol.

Sulphur oxides are of less significance in vehicle emissions than stationary sources, although it is to be noted that they are discharged, as are all other vehicular pollutants, near ground level. Some countries require exhaust catalysts to be installed to burn the hydrocarbon and CO contents of the engine waste gases, and where these are used, some oxidation of SO_2 to SO_3 may take place and lead to the formation of sulphuric acid. SO_2 may also play some part in the oxidation of NO to NO_2 and the subsequent formation of peroxyacetyl nitrate (PAN), a highly irritant gas evolved in photochemical smogs.

Photochemical smog formation is dependant on the presence of primary air pollutants and the climatic conditions of strong sunlight and still air. These conditions are found abundantly in Los Angeles, but many other cities in the world are subject to the same climatic conditions and are on the verge of acquiring the vehicles which will be the primary sources to complete the recipe. The chemistry involved is extremely complicated, but may be considered to be triggered by reservoirs of hydrocarbons, oxidants, and free radicals in the air. Hydrocarbons are provided by the evaporation and incomplete combustion of fuel, oxidants by the action of sunlight on nitrogen oxides, and free radicals by sunlight causing the dissociation of aldehydes (partially oxidized hydrocarbons) into alkyl and formyl (HCO) groups. Chain reactions are liable to perpetuate the cycle by the combination of free radicals with atmospheric oxygen, leading to the production of ozone, thus supplementing the oxidant pool, or with oxygen and NO, leading to the generation of NO_2 and further free radicals. Further reactions produce PAN, acrolein, and the complex mixtures of secondary and subsequent pollutants making up the smog.

In the long term, the control of vehicle emissions is likely to be as much influenced by the price and availability of oil as legislative or technical developments, as more economical use is made of this scarce resource and alternative means of propulsion are sought. Cars fuelled by alcohol derived from sugar cane are already in production, notably in Brazil, and, although costing about 10% more to manufacture and consuming about 10% more fuel, hold out the hope of increasing independance from oil to those countries possessing the land and climate suitable for growing the raw material for alcohol production. As these fuels are virtually pollution-free, they promise the extra bonus of environmental improvement.

8.1.3 Self-imposed air pollution

Self-imposed air pollution cannot escape mention as a significant cause of ill health, occurring primarily from the inhalation of cigarette smoke. Christopher Columbus first observed the smoking of tobacco in the West Indies in 1492. The tobacco habit began to spread to Europe during the sixteenth century, and about 1559, Jean Nicot, the French ambassador in Portugal obtained some seeds and raised the plants in his garden, claiming that tobacco had medicinal properties. He was very much responsible for the popularization of smoking in France, hence the name of the plant species, *Nicotiniana*, and of the principal alkaloid of the plant, nicotine. Sir Walter Raleigh is credited with popularizing pipe smoking in England, for centuries the sole method of smoking tobacco adopted in this country. The cigar became popular on the continent, and English army officers adopted the habit of smoking them during the Peninsular War (1808—14), following which cigars were imported into England, subject to high customs duties. Cigarettes were first brought to England, again by army officers, at the end of the Crimean War (1854—56). Their use quickly became fashionable, and from 1888 onwards the cigarette became increasingly popular and the use of the pipe and cigar began to decline. By 1918, as much tobacco was being used for cigarettes as for pipes, and from then on the pipe rapidly gave way to the cigarette (Fig. 8.3).

In those early days, the smoking of cigarettes was exclusively a male habit and it was not until after the first world war that women began to adopt the practice in significant numbers. The first years in which sales of manufactured cigarettes to women are recorded in the statistics of the Tobacco Research Council is 1921, when women are shown as having consumed 0.6 million pounds manufactured weight by comparison with the 77.5 million pounds manufactured weight of cigarettes consumed by males. It seems probable that some women were smoking cigarettes even before the first world war, and that that this event may have stimulated the spread of the habit amongst them. Over the years, female consumption of cigarettes has tended to lag behind that of men, but nevertheless has continued to show a steady increase even after male consumption had begun to fall (Fig. 8.4).

The later start of cigarette smoking by women may have a particular significance in relation to their delayed experience of the lung cancer epidemic (see p. 59).

The story of the cigarette is not just a matter of historical interest, but also of

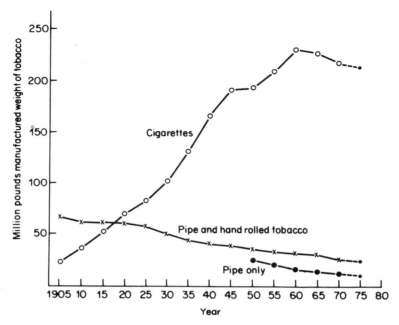

Fig. 8.3   Sales of tobacco goods to the public in the United Kingdom 1905–75. Ten years averages (1975 figure is actual consumption that year). (Data from Tobacco Research Council, 1976.)

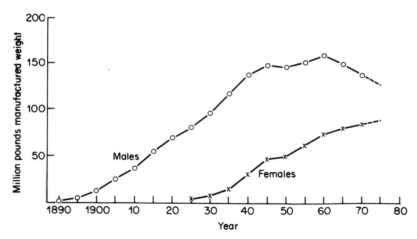

Fig. 8.4   Consumption of manufactured cigarettes in the United Kingdom 1890–1975, by sex. (Data from Tobacco Research Council, 1976.)

considerable present day importance, for it is of significance that the use of tobacco, mainly in the form of cigarettes, is a relatively recent social event in the United Kingdom, dating back only some sixty years. It is a social change which has had untold consequences upon the health of the nation. The smoking of cigarettes is associated with an increased risk of bronchitis (Chap. 6), lung cancer (Chap. 4), and cardiovascular disease (Chap. 5), amounting between them to the most important causes of morbidity and mortality in the country at this time. In their publication *Smoking and Health Now* the Royal College of Physicians estimated that there were some 31 000 premature deaths associated with cigarette smoking amongst men aged 35–64 in the United Kingdom in 1968, and came to the conclusion that at least half of these were actually due to smoking. The report states: 'It would not be unreasonable to attribute to cigarette smoking 90% of the deaths from lung cancer, 75% of those from chronic bronchitis, and 25% of those from coronary artery disease. These probably conservative assumptions lead to an estimate of about 24 000 deaths from these three diseases caused by cigarette smoking among men aged 35–64'. The emphasis here is upon the unnecessarily early deaths of relatively young men who otherwise would have been in their prime. Evidence is now accumulating that even exposure of non-smokers to cigarette smoke generated by others can lead to an increased risk of ill-health. In the light of this self-inflicted pollution of the air which we all must breathe, popular anxieties about the hazards of low levels of lead in the environment, or of the possible risks associated with the release of low level radioactivity from nuclear power stations pale into utter insignificance.

Other instances of self-inflicted ill-health and injury include the inhalation of solvent vapours from adhesives and cleaning fluids, liver damage and death having been recorded as a result. In Australia, gasoline-sniffing has been named as a cause of raised blood-lead levels among less responsible elements of the younger generation.

8.1.4 Indoor air pollution

The significance of indoor air pollution is being increasingly appreciated as energy costs cause more attention to be directed towards draught-proofing and insulation. The effects of tobacco smoke in public buildings, particularly entertainment places, can be readily seen in air conditioning and ventilation plant and ductwork. Recognition that the non-smoker is subject to this form of pollution by passive inhalation is leading to progressively greater restrictions on the use of tobacco in public places. In the home, concentration of nitrogen dioxide from the use of gas cookers has been examined as a potential hazard as the number of hourly air changes is reduced in the interests of energy conservation. The Royal Commission on Environmental Pollution has considered concentrations of radon and its daughter products in buildings, arising from the decay of naturally-occurring radium in building materials and has recommended a maximum acceptable limit of 25mSv annual effective dose equivalent.

8.2 Food

Although a clear understanding of the microbiology and chemistry of food has only been acquired in comparatively recent times, the principles of food hygiene have long been appreciated and applied. The ancient Jews founded the practice of meat inspection and wisely rejected the flesh of any sick or moribund animal as unfit for consumption. Their prohibition of the consumption of pork recognized the risk of contracting the nematode infestation *Trichinella spiralis* from this meat.

Food can be a vehicle for the transmission of pathogenic organisms by both toxic and infective mechanisms. Infective food poisoning, specific food-borne infections and parasitic infestations involving attacks on the body by active hostile agents, are discussed in Chap. 3. Toxic food poisoning occurs when body tissues are subjected to the toxins, or poisonous waste products, arising from the previous multiplication of bacteria in food.

The most common source of toxic food poisoning is the staphylococcus group of organisms, frequently found in abscesses and infected cuts and often carried without apparent ill-effect in the nasal secretions of many people. Given an appropriate high-protein growth medium, such as meat or milk products, and a suitable temperature, 5–60°C, exponential growth takes place, limited only by competition for the available nutrients and the restricting environment of the organisms' own wastes. Once the toxins are produced, they are stable even at temperatures which are high enough to destroy the parent bacteria and may not be broken down even at 100°C. They thus survive cooking processes, as well as refrigeration. This group is a strong candidate for suspicion in any case showing symptoms of abdominal pain, nausea, vomiting and diarrhoea about six hours after ingesting one of the high-risk foods. The condition is very rarely fatal, but risks increase in the young, the aged and those already in poor health.

Poisoning by *Clostridium perfringens* toxin usually takes a mild form with the onset occurring 12–14 hours after ingestion. The organism is a common inhabitant of soil and the digestive tract of man and livestock and there are thus many opportunities for transmission to food during slaughter, processing and preparation, unless proper care in hygiene and temperature storage is exercised.

By far the most serious form of toxic food poisoning of bacterial origin is caused by *Clostridium botulinum* – botulism. The organism is widely distributed in the environment and contamination of raw food is not uncommon, but heat treatment during processing is usually sufficient to kill the bacteria, though not necessarily any spores. Production of the toxin, which is one of the most powerful poisons known, requires a long period of storage under anaerobic conditions with abundant moisture and no more than moderate acidity. Good canning practice will ensure the destruction of *C. botulinum* by holding the entire contents of the can above the organism's thermal death point of 116°C for 10 minutes, or higher temperatures for less time. Cases of botulism, which involve severe and often fatal neurotoxic effects, are generally associated with unsatisfactory home canning techniques. The toxin can, however, be destroyed by subsequent heating.

Moulds grow readily on certain foods and their presence in stale bread is quite familiar. They have largely been regarded as a nuisance, more detrimental to quality than health, but increasing evidence is coming to light that they have adverse effects. *Aspergillus flavus*, affecting certain cereals, produces aflatoxin which has been found to induce changes associated with carcinoma in the liver cells of laboratory animals. Moulds, together with yeasts, are highly resistant to deep-freeze conditions and indicate the need for thorough cleanliness of refrigerators.

Preservation techniques have, from the earliest times, helped to extend the restricted seasonal availability of foods. *Dehydration*, by removing moisture, deprives microorganisms of a pre-requisite to growth, and in early times was accomplished through sun and air. Modern industry makes wide use of accelerated freeze-drying, in which the water content of quickly frozen products is sublimated directly to the vapour state, preserving the cellular structure of the food. *Pickling* in vinegar or brine is a traditional method of creating an environment inhospitable to spoilage and pathogenic organisms. *Pasteurization* involves relatively mild heat treatment of milk and other beverages to destroy likely pathogens and reduce drastically the population of spoilage organisms. *Sterilization*, by employing higher temperatures, greatly extends storage life and the still higher temperatures of *ultra-heat treatment* enable milk to be kept for months without refrigeration. The stabilization of bacterial populations at a low level by *deep-freezing* has been practiced for decades commercially and now finds wide domestic application. *Irradiation* is carried out to inhibit the sprouting of vegetables as well as to destroy pathogenic organisms and insect pests.

These processes may involve some sacrifice in food quality. Deep-frozen products suffer a gradual loss of vitamin C content with time and the temperatures and exposure times used in heat-treatment must be carefully adjusted to prevent deterioration of the flavour, appearance and nutritional content.

These valuable techniques have been supplemented by chemical preservation and further substances have been developed to improve flavour, texture and appearance. Gross adulteration of food for gain is now rare and additions are made on a highly scientific basis. Additives include the following:

Preservatives   e.g. sulphur dioxide, sorbic acid, benzoic acid, sodium nitrate, ascorbic acid;
Emulsifiers   e.g. tartaric acid esters, glycerides, propylene glycol;
Stabilizers   e.g. agar agar, carab gum, cellulose ethers, brominated vegetable oils;
Anti-oxidants   e.g. n-propyl gallate, n-octyl gallate, n-dodecyl gallate, butylated hydroxianisole, butylated hydroxitoluene;
Solvents   e.g. ethyl alcohol, ethyl acetate, glycerol, iso-propyl alcohol;
Colouring matter   e.g. coal tar derivatives, carbon black, iron oxide, caramel, cochineal, annatto;
Flavourings   e.g. vanilla, acetaldehyde, benzaldehyde;
Tenderizers   e.g. proteolytic enzymes, papain;
Sweeteners   e.g. saccharin, saccharin calcium, saccharin sodium.

Some of these are of natural animal or vegetable origin, but the majority are chemically produced to meet the requirements of cost, convenience and consistency.

In view of the potentially serious consequences of using additives, strict control over the nature and amounts has to be exercised. A formidable task faces those charged with the responsibility of setting appropriate limits for the long-term protection of the consumer and much experimental work is necessary, using animal (but see p. 73) and other biological trials, before new additives can safely be allowed on the market. Judgements may then have to be modified in the light of experience gained from monitoring the use of the products over a period of years.

Unintended chemical contamination of food may arrive via the routes of uptake from soil, chemical action on containers, processing plant or packaging materials, accidental adulteration, impurities in process water, or direct contamination from applied treatments or air pollution. Accidental but highly dangerous chemical contamination of food can occur where handling or storage techniques are defective. For example, in Iraq, consumption of seed corn intended for planting, which had been treated with mercury compounds, led to serious toxicological consequences in the victims, and in Colombia spillage of an organochlorine pesticide from a broken bottle contaminated a bag of flour lying in the same railway wagon. The result was a number of deaths after the bakery of a small town unsuspectingly used the flour and distributed loaves prepared from it.

The traditional type of pewter contains a substantial proportion of lead and many drinking vessels still in use provide their users with a small, unnoticed dose of lead additional to intake from other sources. Similar hazards may be attached to the use of ceramic vessels with defective glazed surfaces.

The unceasing quest for increased productivity from land has led to the farm becoming a chemical workshop and materials are in everyday use to control weeds and insect pests and to preserve and enhance the value of livestock. Many common pesticides are recognized as highly toxic and although the world owes much to these substances in the promotion of public health through the control of vector-borne diseases and the protection of vital food crops, residues are commonly to be found in food, where the long-term effects of chronic intake by humans are still not completely understood.

Polychlorinated biphenyls (PCBs), used increasingly since the 1930s as dielectric fluids and in paints, plasticizers and adhesives have caused concern as persistent toxic pollutants in water, and thus food through absorption by fish. The EEC Council requires member states to exercise care over the disposal of material containing PCBs, in view of the risks of water contamination by tip leachate. Unusually high levels have, on occasions, been recorded in fish as a result of local pollution incidents. A study of PCBs, together with metals and organochlorine pesticides in fish and shellfish landed in England and Wales in 1974 concluded that PCB residues were low by all standards of safety but that the distribution of these pollutants required continuing surveillance to maintain safety margins.

The use of hormones and antibiotics has become widespread on account of the benefits to be derived from their application to food animals, where, by altering the synthesis of proteins and fats from fodder and by limiting the growth of debilitating parasitic populations, they promote the efficient conversion of animal food into marketable meat. Careful control of the dose is essential and, with good livestock management, hormones are largely eliminated by the time of slaughter, but, once again, the long-term effects of repeated minute doses are unknown. Antibiotics in milk certainly require strict limitation to prevent ill-effects on consumers who may be sensitized to them and disruption of subsequent microbiological actions in the manufacture of dairy products. Many applications of hormones to plant growth are also in use or under development.

The food chain is an important concept in environmental protection, recognizing that pollutants or additives introduced into the environment at some point may find their way back to man via unintended routes. Thus, for example, drift from herbicides sprayed onto soil may affect nearby grazing pastures and persist in the bodies of cattle, affecting milk and meat at a later stage. In some cases, concentration of substances can occur in intermediate food species and has been studied in chains commencing with aquatic plants, through molluscs to fish and finally to birds preying on the fish, with increasing bodily levels of the substances detected at each link or stage.

8.3   Pure water

The importance of clean water supplies to the health of the community can hardly be overstressed and, worldwide, remains a substantial public health problem.

Obviously, drinking water must be of high quality and present no risks to the consumer by its chemical, biological or microbiological content. Only a small proportion of daily water consumption is attributable to drinking, but personal washing, laundering and food preparation all require pure water supplies for the protection of health. The carriage of sewage, whilst not *per se* requiring high quality water, is another important facet of the relationship of water to health.

Water is constantly in the process of being recycled by nature, evaporation from rivers, lakes and the oceans leading to precipitation and providing fresh distilled supplies to the earth's surface. Bacteria play a key role in breaking down polluting matter and rendering it innocuous and their activities which are undertaken quite naturally in water courses have been harnessed for useful application in a concentrated way in sewage treatment plants. The consumption of water in industrialized countries now amounts to 200—250 l per person per day and, clearly, nature requires some assistance in the purification cycle, faced with the quantity of waste water from both personal and industrial use which this volume of consumption implies.

The manifold sources of water supplies — reservoirs, wells, rivers — are all subject to pollution which must be dealt with before the water is fit for use. Rivers, in particular, may be subject to a lengthy list of possible pollution sources, with wide diversity in the nature of the contaminants (see below).

Industrial waste discharges   Acids, alkalis, metals, salts, product waste, all other forms of chemical pollution, rinse waters, spillages.
Sewage disposal   Suspended/dissolved organic material, inorganic material, microorganisms, detergents, metals.
Tip leachate   Organic material from decomposing matter, dumped materials.
Drainage from surfaces   Grit, oil, tar, spilt chemicals.
Agricultural waste   Organic material, pesticides, fertilizers.
Thermal pollution   Detrimental to the reproduction, growth, freedom of movement and healthiness of fish.

8.3.1   Sewage treatment

The simplest forms of sewage treatment are based on conservancy, i.e. containing and holding effluent whilst bacterial purification takes place. In a cesspit, still in common domestic use in sparsely populated areas, relatively little improvement in effluent quality is achieved and the contents, whilst perhaps suitable for cautious distribution on land in controlled quantities often require chemical disinfection and deodourization before they can be considered suitably treated. The septic tank is a somewhat more sophisticated system, relying on a system of internal baffles to delay the passage of sewage through the structure and encouraging the settlement of solids whilst anaerobic bacteria decompose the organic matter present. Sludge settles at the bottom of the tank, from which it is removed periodically, sufficient being left to act as a reservoir of bacterial activity, and the treated water is discharged, or further purified by biological filtration.

Sewage treatment on a municipal or commercial scale involves the screening of incoming effluent to remove bulky solids, which are either incinerated or returned to the system after maceration. Coarse grit, or detritus, is removed in settlement channels before the sewage is processed through sedimentation tanks which allow finer particles to separate and settle as sludge. The sludge may either be dumped at sea or returned to land after consolidation and dewatering, or after further digestion by anaerobic bacteria in heated chambers, the latter process producing a marketable and inoffensive material. The water remaining after sedimentation may be dealt with by biological filtration or the activated sludge process.

Biological filtration relies on the establishment of colonies of microorganisms on a stable medium having a large surface area per unit volume, such as slag, hard coke or clinker, over which the water is slowly trickled, even and constant distribution usually being accomplished by means of a system of rotating perforated discharge pipes. Slow percolation of the water through the filter bed enables the bacteria to oxidize and stabilize the sewage impurities. A high quality effluent is readily obtained in this way, but further treatment by microfiltration through sand beds may be necessary where standards of quality need to be especially stringent.

The activated sludge process employs the same principle, but the bacteria are cultured in sludge which is mixed continuously for some hours with the settled sewage in the presence of artificially entrained or injected air. When purification is complete, a further period of settlement is necessary to allow separation of the sludge and treated water.

8.3.2 Water for public consumption

The fitness of water supplies for public consumption may be assured by minimal treatment where high-purity sources are available, but otherwise may demand extensive treatment, typically involving the following stages.

(*1*)   Collection of surface water or abstraction from river, followed by coarse screening. Natural purification proceeds in the reservoir by settlement of suspended matter and the action of sunlight. Growth of algae is prevented by copper sulphate addition.

(*2*)   Water pumped to treatment works, filtration through activated carbon to remove taste/odour.

(*3*)   Initial chlorine treatment to control bacteria.

(*4*)   Microstraining, for removal of small suspended particles.

(*5*)   Coagulation, for removal of finer particles, by the use of aluminium sulphate, ferric sulphate or ferric chloride, forming a floc which acts as a filter for the particles.

(*6*)   Filtration. Sand is the basic medium, but several distinct layers of media may be used for improved efficiency and the process may either take place under the influence of gravity only (slow filtration) or under pressure in enclosed vessels (rapid filtration).

(*7*)   Aeration, to replace and introduce oxygen in the water to improve palatability and, to some extent, provide a reserve ready to act on any remaining organic material requiring oxidation.

(*8*)   Disinfection, most commonly by chlorine, the residual dose being controlled by dechlorination to limit any excess concentration at the point of consumption.

The quality of water may be described by reference to its physical, chemical and biological characteristics.

Drinking water must have an acceptable degree of palatability, irrespective of its quality otherwise, and therefore needs to be free from unpleasant taste or odour. Turbidity, or the cloudiness of water, is caused by the presence of suspended solid particles and is another important quality factor.

8.3.3 Chemical quality of water

Unless some specific analysis is required to check the presence of a suspected contaminant, the following properties are usually considered the most significant in describing the chemical quality of water:

(1) pH value
(2) Hardness
(3) Chlorides
(4) Fluorides
(5) Nitrates and nitrites
(6) Phosphates
(7) Chlorine

(8) Total organic carbon
(9) Biological Oxygen Demand (BOD)
(10) Ammonia
(11) Sulphide
(12) Detergents
(13) Salinity
(14) Heavy metals

In pure water at 25°C the number of hydrogen (H^+) and hydroxyl (OH^-) ions is equal and the *pH value*, defined as the negative logarithm (to base 10) of the hydrogen ion concentration, is 7. A lowering of this value represents acidity and its elevation towards the limit of 14 is indicative of increasing alkalinity. In either case, a significant departure from the neutral value demonstrates the presence of a chemical state inconsistent with pure water, without necessarily implying any toxic property, unless, of course, the water is grossly acidic or alkaline. The potency of certain pollutants in water may vary with differing pH values.

Hardness is a property affecting the lathering properties of soaps and is due to calcium, magnesium and iron salts dissolved during the percolation of water over and through strata containing these substances. The carbonate salts are mainly insoluble and are precipitated on heating the water, contributing to scale in pipes and vessels (temporary hardness). The sulphate or chloride salts are not removed in this way (permanent hardness). Magnesium and calcium as elements may be of interest in view of their relationship to hardness and calcium may be of significance in the corrosive properties of the water. The association between water hardness and decreased incidence of cardiovascular mortality is considered in Chap. 5 (p. 88).

Chlorides, whilst of low toxicity, may be an indicator of sewage pollution and, taken with other chemical characteristics, can be helpful in classifying an unknown source.

Fluorides occur naturally in many areas and are added to some public water supplies, since at 1 p.p.m. they have been found to cause a significant reduction in the incidence of dental caries. At high levels, fluorides are responsible for staining and mottling of tooth enamel and are thus undesirable.

As *nitrates* are derived from the natural decay of organic matter, they may be indicative of sewage or other pollution. They are also found in watercourses as a result of the use of fertilizers on land. Nitrates are implicated in methaemoglobinaemia ('blue-baby' disease) by conversion to *nitrites* in the low-acid environment of the infant digestive tract and interference with oxygen absorption by the blood, and may be ingested either by high-nitrate waters being used to make up feeds or indirectly via the breast milk of a mother who has been drinking such water. European standards limit nitrate concentration to 50 p.p.m. These compounds must also be considered in the light of research which has shown nitrosamines, produced by bacterial action on nitrates in the intestine, to be carcinogenic in animals, though nitrates and nitrites also occur in certain cured foods as well as water and their effect on adults has not yet been fully researched.

Phosphates supply nutrient to aquatic plants. Their presence is important since excessive plant growth may lead to depletion of dissolved oxygen during their phase of oxygen consumption at night, with consequent suffocation of fish. This process is known as eutrophication (see Barrington, 1980).

Chlorine, despite the development of ozone treatment processes, still plays an important part in the disinfection of potable and swimming bath waters (see Chap. 10) and analysis of total and free chlorine is important in assessing the amount of residual protection at the point of consumption or exposure.

Total organic carbon is normally found at the 2–3 p.p.m. level in drinking water. Unusually high levels may indicate organic pollution, being particularly important where tip leachate is suspected as a cause of contamination, and indicating the need for more specific investigations where the content increases in one of a series of samples.

Biological Oxygen Demand (BOD) gives an important index of overall water quality by measuring the amount of oxygen required by bacteria in breaking down organic matter and hence the degree of organic pollution present. BOD is defined as the weight of oxygen consumed by one litre of water when stored in darkness at $20°C$ for five days. A typical value for raw domestic sewage would be 250 mgl^{-1} and for a clean river, 0.0025 mg l^{-1}. It is usually helpful to know the dissolved oxygen content in conjuction with BOD.

Ammonia and its salts in solution indicate the presence of decomposing matter and are thus a warning of possible sewage contamination. Somewhat elevated concentrations of abuminoid ammonia may be found in peaty waters, through the decomposition of nitrogenous substances, but high ammonia levels of whatever type must always be regarded with suspicion.

Sulphide estimations are normally required only where some unpleasant odour suggests the necessity for more detailed investigation.

Detergents may be present through untreated or insufficiently treated effluent and are thus significant as an indicator of pollution. They may give rise to foaming, taste or toxicity problems.

High *salinity* may create a hostile environment for aquatic life, as well as increasing the corrosive properties of the water.

Metals and their compounds are frequently poisonous to fish, plant life and humans, although trace concentrations of many metals are essential to life. Lead is particularly significant as a human health risk where soft, acidic water has been in contact with lead pipes for any appreciable time before drawing off, and may reach concentrations in excess of the maximum of 50 $\mu g\ l^{-1}$ in water proposed as an EEC standard (see p. 120). Cadmium, copper, zinc, mercury, nickel and chromium may also be hazardous in excessive concentrations.

8.3.4   Microbial quality of water

Many forms of pathogenic microorganisms can be found in polluted water. Cholera, typhoid fever, paratyphoid fever and dysentery are recognized water-borne diseases. The causative organisms of anthrax, brucellosis, tuberculosis, leptospirosis and poliomyelitis can all travel in sewage and there is a suspicion that they may be transmitted in this way.

A valuable tracer and indicator of sewage pollution is *Escherichia coli*, found abundantly in the faeces of humans and other animals. Strains of this organism are believed to be pathogenic to children, but the group, as a whole, is usually regarded as being a relatively minor health risk. In faecal matter numbers of *E. coli* normally exceed those of pathogenic organisms by a very large margin, and a water low in *E. coli* is thus likely to be completely free of harmful bacteria, certainly at any concentration likely to produce disease. Related coliform organisms are also indicative of pollution, not necessarily faecal in origin.

Whilst in ideal circumstances public water supplies should be free of all coliform bacteria, standards allow some flexibility. The World Health Organization recommends an upper limit of 50 coliform bacteria per 100 ml in raw waters intended for distribution after disinfection only. Sources containing 50–5000 are only regarded suitable for use if treated by the conventional processes of coagulation and filtration followed by disinfection. More heavily contaminated waters are only acceptable if much more rigorous treatment is to be applied and at levels over 50 000 the water should only be used where unavoidable and then only after special treatment.

These quality controls are designed to ensure that the water, after treatment, will be suitable for public consumption, i.e. totally free of *E. coli*, with 95% of samples free of any coliform organisms and coliform organisms never present in any two consecutive samples or in greater concentration than 10 per 100 ml.

The biological nature of water is important, both as an indicator of pollution demonstrated by the species which can tolerate that environment and in terms of harmful agents which may be present. In the purest rivers, high levels of dissolved oxygen enable trout and salmon to prosper, but in slightly polluted water their place may be taken by chub and dace, with roach and gudgeon present as the concentration of organic material increases until the point is reached where fish life disappears. Smaller organisms will also vary as organic material rises, caddis and mayflies giving way to freshwater molluscs and snails, then leeches, followed by bloodworms, until, in a highly polluted environment, sewage fungus and sewage worms may be the predominant form of life. A biological assay is thus a helpful guide in assessing the overall quality of water courses.

Some 200 million people, mainly in tropical regions, suffer from the debilitating and unpleasant water-borne infestation by trematode worms known as schistosomiasis. The transmission of this condition is dependant on a cycle involving the penetration of snail hosts by the miracidium from mature eggs contained in excreta hatching on contact with water. Multiplication takes place within the snail over a period of weeks and cercariae are released which penetrate the human skin and develop into adult worms in the blood vessels of the abdominal cacity. From this point eggs are laid which pass into the intestine and bladder, to be excreted and complete the cycle.

8.4 Relationship between air, food, water and land

A review of the hazards liable to be present in air, food and water would be incomplete without reference to the relationships which exist between them, often involving the medium of land. Air pollution, for instance, can lead to fall-out on land making it unsuitable for crop or livestock production. This effect has been noted in connection with the smelting and refining of metals. In the Far East, agricultural work poses threats not only to the workers employed in rice fields flooded with sewage contaminated water, from parasitic conditions, but to the crops themselves from bacillary infection, which may survive through to the point of consumption.

Over 40% of the treated sewage sludge produced in Britain is deposited on land for agricultural purposes, because of its valuable content of the plant nutrients nitrogen and phosphorus and role as a soil conditioner. The metal content of soils treated in this way requires careful long-term monitoring because of their phytotoxicity and the need to prevent undue accumulation (particularly of cadmium) and introduction into the food chain. Complete elimination of disease producing organisms is not guaranteed by sewage treatment and, whilst direct links between sludge disposal and human disease are not totally established, regard must be paid to the possible risks of direct contact and the contamination of water courses by run-off from the land. Much more positive evidence exists to link the transmission of parasitic conditions in this way because of the vast numbers of eggs excreted by infected humans, and their resistance to hostile environments. Sewage sludge is a proven vehicle in the cycle of the bovine infestation cysticercosis.

The redevelopment of land used formerly for industry or waste disposal and now increasingly in demand for residential and commercial occupation poses many practical, environmental and economic problems. Particular difficulties arise with gas works sites, where coal tar derivatives, cyanide, hydrogen sulphide and arsenic are some of the hazards which may be encountered on disturbance of the ground. Sites made up with tipped asbestos waste or furnace residues containing toxic materials are also a major problem. The assessment of contaminated sites must be based on analysis following careful core-sampling at representative points, which may need to be large in number if the waste is mixed or has been deposited in layers or pockets.

The health of construction workers and the future occupants of the land, especially children, requires careful protection, together with preventing the distribution of particulates during the stripping and transport of the contaminated soil and its disposal elsewhere. In some cases, a whole site may have to be excavated and new soil imported, involving a tremendous removal operation. In others, it may be more practicable to cover the contaminated material to a depth of up to 2 m with layered material designed to prevent the upward migration of toxic chemicals. Extra costs in building foundation construction are usual in either case. In some situations, the hazardous material can be encapsulated by building design incorporating large areas of impermeable surface cover, such as car parks or piazzas. Choice of site may be dictated by the avoidance of vulnerable types of development, such as food processing or residential.

Pollution control itself may be a polluting activity. Where air pollution has been abated by wet-scrubbing methods, a liquid waste product requires disposal. This may not be an easy problem to deal with if particulates with a toxic content have been collected in this way and secondary pollution of water or land is to be prevented. Attempts to control sulphur dioxide emissions by scrubbing with chalk-bearing water have been effective, but only at the cost of oxygen depletion from the water and the production of another waste product, calcium sulphate. The process has been found to produce a net overall benefit to the environment in only a few special situations.

Direct contamination of water and food may arise from air pollution. The increase in total emissions of sulphur dioxide to the air over the period 1870—1970 is estimated to be almost twenty-fold. Whilst the more extreme claims about the effects of the international transport of this gas are, perhaps, exaggerated, effects on the acidity of lakes through dissolution of SO_2 in rainwater cannot be dismissed.

care to be taken over the ventilation of premises to prevent the introduction of airborne contaminants into manufacturing areas.

If the environment is regarded as a unified system, no form of pollution can be viewed in isolation. The Royal Commission on Environmental Pollution (Fifth Report, *Air Pollution Control: An Integrated Approach*) recommended the target of 'best practicable environmental option' as a means of ensuring the minimum adverse impact of industrial processes on our surroundings. Sewage treatment is an abundant source of methane, useful as a pollution-free fuel. The needs of industry for water can be met by the juxtaposition of the consumers and sewage treatment works, the effluent from which, though not treated to potable standards, is an economical alternative to public supplies for cooling purposes. Refuse incineration presents useful opportunities for energy production as well as reducing the bulk and putrescible nature of waste. The view that the total environment must be understood and treated in a comprehensive way finds increasing acceptance and may provide grounds for cautious optimism for the future.

9
Technology – noise and radiation

The benefits of the industrial society include the availability of consumer goods, personal mobility and opportunities to enjoy leisure. The price of these is not to be measured solely in terms of money — against them must be balanced the problems of pollution, noise and the consumption of finite energy and raw material resources. Technology embraces many fields which are considered in this book. Noise and radiation as they affect the community are discussed together in this chapter as factors of a physical nature influencing the environment.

9.1 Noise – nature and measurement

The perception of sound results from waves of fluctuating pressure in an elastic medium which stimulate the hearing mechanisms of the ear and brain. It is a primary means of communication and a source of pleasure where the sounds received convey a welcome message or are arranged in harmonic tones which are musical. Noise can be described as waste or unwanted sound and includes not only displeasing random signals, but sound which at other times or in other places may be desirable. The important characteristics of sound are *amplitude* and *frequency*.

Every sound source emits power which, passing through a unit area in space, creates acoustic intensity, in a range from about $0.001 \, \mu W \, m^{-2}$ produced by a very soft whisper to $10\,000 \, W \, m^{-2}$ or more from a jet engine. This lengthy scale is conveniently expressed in terms of logarithmic increments above a reference level, customarily $10^{-12} \, W$ in acoustics:

$$\text{Sound power level} \, (L_w) \; = \; 10 \log_{10} \frac{W_1}{W_0} \qquad (1)$$

where W_1 is the power emitted and W_0 is the reference level, $10^{-12} \, W$.

L_w is a necessary quantity in acoustic calculations and engineering, since it is fixed, independent of the acoustic environment and a function of the source only. However, as far as the recipient is concerned sound is experienced at the point of perception as *pressure* rather than *power*, and this depends on factors such as distance, impedance of the transmitting medium, reflection, absorption and shielding. The range of values encountered when dealing with sound pressures is also wide, with a factor of about $10^7 : 1$ between the thresholds of hearing ($\sim 2 \times 10^{-5} \, N \, m^{-2}$) and pain ($\sim 200 \, N \, m^{-2}$) and this also is better expressed using a logarithmic scale. Sound power varies as sound pressure squared and a convenient scale is defined as

$$\text{Sound pressure level (L}_p) = 10 \log_{10}\left(\frac{P_1}{P_0}\right)^2$$

$$= 20 \log_{10}\frac{P_1}{P_0} \qquad (2)$$

where P_0 is the reference level, $2 \times 10^{-5}\,\text{N m}^{-2}$.

The relationship between L_w and L_p can be shown mathematically but in practice is likely to be complicated by directional factors inherent in most noise sources and their position in relation to reflecting surfaces, for which corrections must be applied.

The use of logarithmic scales in noise measurement makes arithmetic addition of decibel values inappropriate. For instance, taking an existing sound source and adding an identical one results in a doubling of the quantity W_1/W_0 in equation (1) and L_w is increased by $10 \log_{10} 2 = 10 \times 0.301 \simeq 3\,\text{dB}$ as a consequence. It also happens that the ear displays a logarithmic rather than linear response to sound pressure and an increase of about 10 dB in L_p, i.e. an increase of $\sqrt{10}$ (or 3.16) times, will be experienced as an approximate doubling of loudness. Any increase below 3 dB will be imperceptible. The relationship between acoustic quantities and everyday sounds is shown in Table 9.1.

Table 9.1 Acoustic intensities, pressures and levels compared with everyday sounds.

Intensity (W m^{-2})	Sound pressure (N m^{-2})	Sound pressure level, L_p (db)	Examples
100	200	140	Jet engine at take-off
10	63.24555	130	
1	20	120	
0.1	6.32455	110	Pop concert/large orchestra
0.01	2	100	Woodworking machinery
0.001	0.63245	90	Heavy goods vehicle at kerbside
0.0001	0.2	80	Telephone bell at 1m
0.00001	0.06324	70	Typing at 1m
0.000001	0.02	60	Normal conversation at 1m
0.0000001	0.00632	50	General office
0.00000001	0.002	40	Quiet office
0.000000001	0.00063	30	Interior of country church
0.0000000001	0.0002	20	Broadcasting studio
0.00000000001	0.00006	10	Anechoic chamber
0.000000000001	0.00002	0	Threshold of hearing

Frequency of perceived sound is very important, since the hearing does not respond equally to all noises of a given amplitude if their frequencies differ. Contours of equal loudness, plotted by averaging the results of many subjective assessments in experimental work, demonstrate the nature of the response and the way it varies at different levels of sound (Fig. 9.1).

Measurement of sound enables levels to be compared with standards, where available; it helps in identifying frequency components which are the cause of annoyance and it quantifies the effectiveness of attenuation measures. The sound

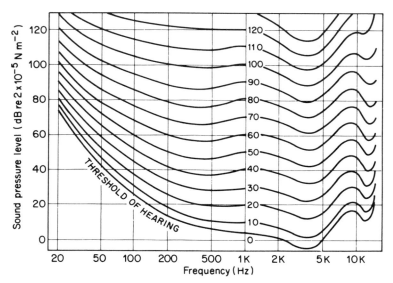

Fig. 9.1 Contours of equal loudness for pure tones (phon curves). (After BS 3383 (ISO R226).)

level meter consists basically of a microphone, preamplifier, one or more amplifiers and an indicating mechanism. To this may be added facilities for frequency analysis and statistical recording capabilities to show the variation of noise with time. Integrating meters are available to represent varying sound over a period in terms of the average energy content of signals per unit of time. The incorporation of chart recorders, tape recorders and digital printers enables a comprehensive record of observations to be kept and modern data capture and processing methods enable very speedy and detailed analyses to be carried out.

Because of the varying response of the ear to differing frequencies of sound, little is to be gained by simply measuring the pressure level indiscriminately over the whole frequency spectrum and expecting the result to correlate with any standard of annoyance or disturbance. For this reason, measurements and standards are usually expressed in weighted form. International standards have been developed to specify 'A', 'B', 'C', and 'D' weightings, as shown in Fig. 9.2.

Comparison with Fig. 9.1 shows that the 'A' weighting curve approximates in shape to the 40 phon contour of equal loudness and this measurement has been found to correlate well with subjective assessments of the loudness of a noise source. 'B' and 'C' weightings follow the general form of the 70 and 100 phon curves, but are not widely used in practice. 'D' weighting has found application in aircraft noise measurement through the addition of amplification at a maximum at 4 KHz to allow for the intrusive component in jet engine noise present at about that frequency. Further weightings have been proposed, namely 'E' and 'S1', being claimed to provide closer correlation with *perceived noisiness* and *speech interference,* respectively. 'A' weighting remains, however, the most widely used.

A single measurement of noise, with whatever weighting, is often insufficient

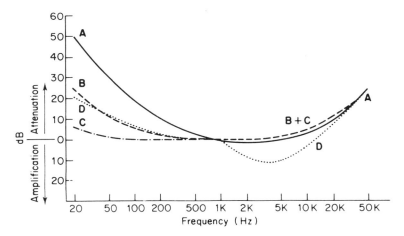

Fig. 9.2 Response of sound level meter with A, B, C, and D weighting filters. (After BS4197 (IEC 179).)

to indicate all the components, especially pure tones, which influence its potential for annoyance or harmfulness. In such cases, the first procedure may be to carry out analysis in octave bands. The preferred frequencies are set out in ISO Recommendation R266:1962 and British Standard 3593:1963, namely, octave bands having the geometric centre frequencies of 16, 31.5, 63, 125, 250, 500, 1000, 2000, 4000, 8000 and 16000 Hz. The width of an octave band is defined by the limits $f/\sqrt{2} \rightarrow 2f/\sqrt{2}$, where f is the centre frequency. Thus, the 1000 Hz band covers the range 707–1414 Hz, the 2000 Hz band 1414–2828 Hz, and so on.

Octave band analysis enables the spectrum to be compared with Noise Rating (NR) curves, defined in ISO Recommendation R1996, *Assessment of Noise with Respect to Community Response*. Each curve is numbered according to the level of its intersection of the 1000 Hz ordinate (Fig. 9.3). NR curves enable the noise to be rated by the highest curve into which the measured spectrum intrudes. The example given shows the spectrum from a word processor in a general office, rated at NR 68 at 1 m distance. It can be seen that the highest L_p occurs in the band centred on 63 Hz, but this level of 72 dB only corresponds with NR 45. It is the levels at 1 KHz and 4 KHz which elevate the spectrum to NR 68 and which need reduction, together with the 2 KHz centred band, if a subjective improvement is to be achieved.

More detailed analysis can be carried out, if necessary, in one-third octave bands, narrow bandwidths (e.g. 3 Hz, 10 Hz) or narrow percentage bandwidths (e.g. 3%, 10%) through the spectrum. Each stage of increased detail implies the use of more sophisticated equipment and extra time for analysis, but may prove necessary in identifying the exact frequency which is causing the problem, as attenuation measures must usually be engineered for maximum performance in a closely defined range.

In many situations scales or indices which represent noise events, or the variation of a noise climate with time, form the basis of assessing nuisances and defining standards applicable to their control. Statistical analysis of fluctuating

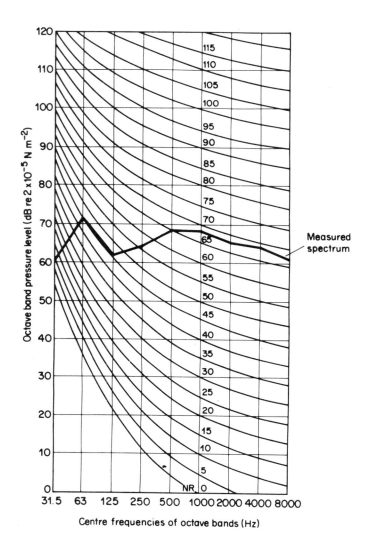

Centre frequencies of octave bands (Hz)

Fig. 9.3   Noise rating curves, with an example spectrum (word processor at 1 m). (After ISO R1996, reproduced by permission of ISO.)

noise over a period is undertaken by examining samples from continuous measurement. The index L_N represents the noise level, usually in dB(A), exceeded for N% of the measurement period. The annoyance due to road traffic has been found to correlate well with the average of hourly L_{10} measurements taken between 0600 hours and the midnight and the L_{10} (18 hour) index has been adopted in the U.K. for the assessment of eligibility for compensation of certain householders adversely affected by the noise from new or altered highways. L_{90} or L_{95} can be taken to represent background noise and, with other statistical indices, have been incorporated into standards for rating industrial noise.

In the search for a unified system of measurement which should predict a general potential for annoyance in an average population, Leq has won support from a number of acousticians because of its relative simplicity and flexibility, despite difficulties in allowing for the disturbance effects of short-duration noises in long measurement periods and the lack of differentiation between day and night times in this composite scale. Leq is effectively a logarithmic average of noise, or a notional steady sound level which would cause the same energy to be received over a period as that actually received.

L_{NP}, the noise pollution level, has been developed from Leq to give a better indication of the nuisance value of successive fluctuating noises. It is defined as

$$L_{NP} = Leq + k\sigma$$

where σ is the standard deviation of the instantaneous sound levels and k is a constant, value 2.56, chosen by subjective studies. This scale includes an element of 'penalty' related to the variability of a sequence of noises.

The Day-Night Average Sound Level, L_{dn} (18), proposed by the United States Environmental Protection Agency is a derivation of Leq, in which a 10 db penalty is applied to noise occurring within the period 2200−0700 hours.

Special consideration has been given to aircraft noise which, unlike that from industry or road traffic is characterized by its periodical, rather than continuous but fluctuating nature. The Noise and Number Index (NNI) was derived from social surveys conducted in the region of London's Heathrow Airport and combines the effect of both the noisiness of individual aircraft and the number of flights in a daytime period. The index introduces the concept of perceived noisiness (PN) expressed in terms of PNdB by weighting the sound pressure level in particular frequency bands and is expressed by

$$NNI = \bar{L}_{PN_{max}} + 15\log_{10}N - 80$$

where $\bar{L}_{PN_{max}}$ is the logarithmic average of the maximum perceived noise levels in PNdB during the passage of successive aircraft and N is the number of movements heard between the hours of 0600 and 1800. Traffic movements accounting for levels below 80 PNdB at the receiving position are left out of account. International Standards Organization publication 3891:1978, adopted as British Standard 5727:1979, prescribes a method for describing aircraft noise heard on the ground and specifies methods for data acquisition, processing, normalization and reporting. It is directed to the characterization of single aircraft movements, in flight or on the ground, and the effects of a succession of these events and employs the quantities of L_{PN} (perceived noise levels), L_{TPN} (tone-corrected perceived noise levels), L_{EPN} (effective perceived noise levels), L_{AX} (single event exposure levels) and L_{PNeq} (equivalent continuous value of L_{PN}).

L_{AX}, the single event noise exposure level, is of interest as a special case of Leq, being defined as the level which, if maintained constant for a period of one second, would cause the same A-weighted sound energy to be received as is actually received from a specific single event.

9.2   Industrial noise

Noise sources in industry may be broadly classified as follows:

Impact   machinery to workpiece, e.g. hammering, forging, saw teeth on material, riveting;
Vibratory   out-of-balance forces in machinery;
Aerodynamic   jets, fans, explosions, exhausts;
Electromagnetic   distortion of motor components subject to changing magnetic fields.

Machinery is, in fact, very inefficient at radiating noise, since acoustic impedance allows limited energy to pass from solid objects into air. Nevertheless, even the very small proportion of total energy which is converted into noise can be enough to cause difficult problems, which are compounded through the effects of amplification and resonance. A simple illustration may be obtained by striking a tuning fork – itself an object designed to be highly resonant at a precise frequency – and holding the handle against a relatively stiff, massive object, such as a bench. The sound will at once increase as the vibration from the fork is efficiently conducted into and through the bench, to be radiated with increased intensity from its large surfaces. Should the bench happen to possess a natural resonant frequency coinciding with that of the tuning fork, the amplification will be further increased.

The control of noise at source through the design of quiet machines is a very desirable objective, but implies a considerable commitment of effort and money. It may well involve the construction of prototype machines to enable detailed noise analysis to be undertaken in the search for offending frequencies, which are likely to increase in number with the complexities of the physical structure and the presence of harmonics, presenting time-consuming diagnostic problems. Attempts to design out the offending frequencies may well be frustrated by the creation of a new spectrum of sound from altered components. Where mass and stiffness of the structural parts are altered in the interests of noise control, weight and cost penalties may soon be subject to a law of diminishing returns. Cheap and effective engineering methods are, fortunately, applicable to some situations. For instance, amplification can be prevented by isolating vibrating parts from panels, using insulators of the correct materials and dimensions to suit the frequency characteristics and size of the noise source. Noise radiated from panels can be greatly reduced by constructional use of steel damped by a surface coating or 'sandwich' of damping material between two metal skins.

Where reduction at source has been taken to its economic limit, it may be necessary to separate the noise producer and receiver by either physical barriers or distance. This can be achieved by enclosing the noisiest machines, as long as the needs of access and ventilation can be met, or the sound insulation of buildings may need to be improved for the protection of the neighbouring community. Where these measures are, for some reason impracticable, separation of source and receiver may be the only answer, by the relocation of either. Sound from a point source decreases by 6dB with each doubling of distance and extra losses arise due to the impedance of air (of noticeable value only at higher frequencies) and absorption by intervening ground or vegetation. These effects may be enhanced or frustrated by prevailing climatic conditions.

Duration of noise is also an important factor and British and international standards for rating the nuisance value of industrial noise make allowances for 'on-time', as well as irregularities in its character and the presence of any distinguishable note.

Some indication of the relative importance of industrial noise *vis-à-vis* other sources can be gained from the number of complaints made to Environmental Health Officers in England and Wales over the years (Fig. 9.4). Complaints received are not a perfect measure of the size of any problem, but these figures show that although the overall number of cases has tended to increase slightly, the proportion of complaints directed towards industry has declined from over 40% to about 20% in eight years whilst other sources, particularly domestic premises have featured much more prominently.

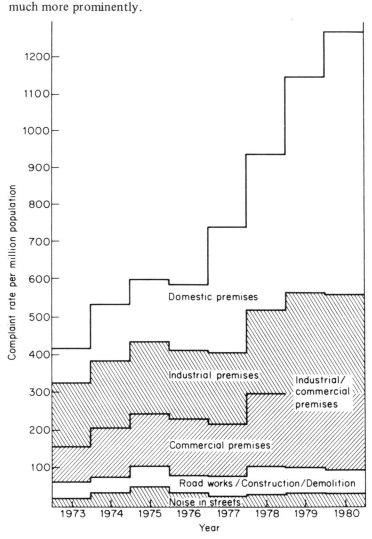

Fig. 9.4 Trends in noise complaints received by environmental health officers in England and Wales. Complaint rates per million persons.(From Department of the Environment, *Digest of Environmental Pollution and Water Statistics*. No. 4, (1981). H.M.S.O.)

9.3   Transport noise

Road traffic noise is a widely experienced problem, without straightforward means of alleviation except in very specialized situations. Regulations made under the Land Compensation Act, 1973, provide that the highway authority must bear the cost of sound insulation of nearby houses subject to increased noise from new or altered highways where the resulting level is over L_{10} (18-hour) 68dB(A) (see p. 140), but this provision is, of course, without value to the receivers of noise from existing roads caused by the gradual increase of traffic over the years. Dissatisfaction in these circumstances has created strong public pressures for the construction of relief roads and the effect of these has been dramatic in restoring quality to the environment of many communities.

Where social surveys have been undertaken, it has emerged that road traffic noise is the principal and most widespread source of annoyance to the general public. One estimate places the number of U.K. citizens exposed to traffic noise of L_{10} (18-hour) 70 dB(A) or greater at 14 millions in 1980 – a 64% increase compared with 1970. Where traffic flows, and thus L_{10} (18-hour) noise levels, are low, the noise from individual motorcycles is frequently quoted as the predominant source of annoyance.

Vehicle noise arises principally from the engine and mechanical components, including the cooling fan, and from tyres and exhaust systems. These factors assume varying significance according to speed, congestion, gradients and road surfaces (particularly if wet).

Road design is an important factor in mitigating the effects of traffic noise. Distance attenuation, cuttings and barriers all have their part to play in reducing propagation. A doubling of distance from a 'line' source, for example, a road, results in a reduction of some 3dB where the intervening ground is reflective, or about 4dB over grassland. The attenuation achieved by noise screens and landscaping measures is examined at length in the Department of Environment book, *Calculation of Road Traffic Noise* (1976).

Progress in the design of quieter vehicles is, in the long-term, expected to provide some relief as long as traffic flows do not increase and thus negate this benefit, but it will take many years for the effect to spread throughout the total vehicle population. As tyre noise tends to predominate at high speeds, this may mask the benefits obtained from quieter engines and exhaust systems.

Aircraft noise imposes a considerable burden on the community in terms of lowered amenity and property values. Some relief from the noisier jet aircraft introduced in the 1950s has been gained by engine modifications in which attention has been paid to air velocities, fan speeds, noise absorbers and deflectors, designed to reduce external noise propagation.

Technical noise abatement measures have been matched by a range of operational procedures to reduce nuisance, including the following:

(*i*) *Preferential runway systems* – directing take-offs over less densely populated areas where wind conditions permit.

(*ii*) *Minimum noise routes* – channelling traffic so as to affect the least number of of people. Here a conflict exists between spreading flights over a wide area and concentrating them in narrow air corridors whereby a smaller population is exposed to much more frequent annoyance.

(*iii*) *Take-off noise procedures* – full power/rapid climb on immediate take-off, reduced power over residential areas, then full power to cruising altitude. The reduced power phase may disturb more people and for a longer period, despite the lowering of noise intensity.

(*iv*) *Mufflers and earth banks* into which jet exhausts are directed to absorb noise during taxiing, idling and test running.

(*v*) *Approach paths* — steepening to 3° instead of the preferred 2½° maintains altitude a little longer, with some beneficial effect on noise levels on the ground.

Land use is a key factor in many noise problems and no more so than in the case of siting new or extended airports. Britain is a small country with limited scope for siting airports away from urban areas and, compared with the United States, aircraft are estimated to cause much more annoyance per passenger mile. Planning authorities in England and Wales are advised not to permit development which will involve housing being subjected to 40 NNI or greater and more stringent criteria may be applied to certain rural areas. The Greater London Council, whilst accepting that a more generally applicable index than NNI needs to be developed in the future, has adopted a policy of regarding land within a 60 NNI contour as being definitely unsuitable for dwellings, even with sound insulation.

Subjective assessment of railway noise appears to indicate that it is found less annoying than similar levels from other transport sources. One possible explanation is that mankind has learned to live with railways for a fairly extended period and attitudes to road and air traffic noise might possibly become more accommodating after a longer period of adaptation. The 24 hour Leq scale has been found to be most appropriate for rating railway noise and at Leq 74 this source is only experienced as annoying as other sources having levels some 6–10 dB lower. As might be expected, proximity to the track is a significant factor and new home occupiers are more sensitive. Overhead electric routes are less liable to provoke complaints than third-rail and diesel routes. It is estimated that up to 80 000 homes in Britain could be subject to Leq 65 dB(A) or greater and the problem is likely to grow as railway land in urban areas is increasingly redeveloped for housing purposes. The Greater London Council guidelines require sound insulation for new housing exposed to this level and offer of acquisition of existing housing newly affected by railway noise of Leq 80 dB(A).

9.4   Effects of noise

Noise is discussed in Chapters 10 and 11 as a potential hazard to physical health. There is clear evidence that levels in excess of 90 dB(A) received over an extended period are injurious to hearing and damage may be sustained much earlier at higher levels. Community noise is rarely concerned with such high levels and its effects must be studied in terms of comfort, amenity and annoyance. These are vague terms and objective definition is difficult. Adverse effects can usually be taken to include mental unease, and psychosomatic disturbances such as fatigue, shortness of temper, insomnia and headaches.

Individual reactions vary considerably and mental attitude to the nature of the source as well as the physical features of the noise, seems to be an important factor. To many people, noise from some socially useful activity is likely to be more acceptable than that which they consider to be unnecessary or emanating from a source of which they disapprove. For example, construction noise can be a source of extreme nuisance during particularly active phases of the work, but there is every possibility that complaints will be less if a positive public relations policy is adopted by the developer. Local residents are likely to be much more sympathetic if they are warned in advance of unusually noisy operations and given a chance to reduce disturbance, as far as possible, by negotiating limits on working times to fit in with their own patterns of children's bedtime or shift-workers' rest periods.

Subjective reactions to various sources of noise were examined by the Department of Behavioural Studies, Newcastle-upon-Tyne Polytechnic in 1976. The opinions of residents, published in the report *Noise in Darlington*, are shown in Table 9.2.

Table 9.2   Residents of Darlington, U.K., hearing, and bothered by, various noise sources. (From ***Noise in Darlington***, Department of Behavioural Studies, Newcastle upon Tyne Polytechnic. By courtesy of Victor Jupp, The Open University.)

Noise source	% Hearing	% Bothered
Aircraft	70.4	4.7
Traffic	79.6	20.9
Factories	15.2	4.5
Construction	15	4.3
Animals/birds	81.8	9.1
People/children outside	81.6	14.6
Railways	33.6	3.6

An easily recognized effect of noise is disturbance of sleep. Sleep is an essential period of refreshment, accounting for some one-third of adult existence, and deprivation is a well-known method of applying deliberate psychological pressure to, say, prisoners during 'third-degree' interrogation, weakening the resolve of the subject and impairing his judgement. The same effects may unintentionally result from environmental noise and may occur without the sleeping person necessarily having been awakened. Sleep comprises a number of recognizable stages and levels and elevating a person from deep sleep to a state nearer wakefulness, which may happen through fairly moderate levels of noise, can be just as harmful as total awakening. The elderly are much more easily disturbed or wakened in this way than are children, and women appear to be a little more susceptible than men. In adults, a short duration noise 20dB above background may interfere with deep sleep and a 70dB sound persisting for only one-third of a second may do the same.

People adapt to noise in many circumstances and may be ill at ease in the absence of familiar background sounds, as, for instance, the city-dweller newly removed to the country. Fatigue is commonly associated with noise, yet in some instances, people already tired through loss of sleep caused by exposure to noise may be brought to a higher level of arousal on entering a noisy environment.

As loud and startling noises can produce physiological reactions very similar to those of fear (although these reactions are much reduced on repetitions of the event) it does not seem unreasonable to infer that they are detrimental to health, since fear can hardly be described as a healthy condition. Stress, much criticized as an adverse factor in life and blamed as a contributor to a variety of illnesses, has often been associated with noise. Caution must be exercised in categorizing this as a completely bad effect, as the line between healthy stimulation and unhealthy stress is not easy to draw. What may be stress to one person at one time can easily be stimulation to another at a different time.

Numerous claims, some hardly more than suspicions, have been made about the effects of noise on mental health, but conclusive results have been difficult to obtain from field studies. No doubt, a lot of the effects are not quantifiable in a specific way as there are no precise indices to measure irritability, discomfort and mental unease in people. This does not alter the fact that noise is perceived by a substantial proportion of the population as a serious problem affecting their daily lives and its treatment and minimization are significant economic factors in airport development, vehicle design, civil engineering operations, road planning and public administration. Proof beyond reasonable doubt may not be available, but the circumstantial evidence prompts some disturbing questions:

What part does noise play with other stress factors in the creation of alcohol and drug dependency problems?

How many traffic accidents are caused through noise-induced fatigue?

How many violent crimes (particularly assaults on infants) are precipitated by noise?

How many accidents at work and leisure are occasioned by noise interfering with communications?

What contribution does noise make to absenteeism from work?

9.5   Ionizing radiation

Ionizing radiation is discussed as an occupational hazard in Chapter 11, but deserves consideration in a general environmental context, in view of the greatly increased use of radioactive materials since 1945, for both peaceful and military purposes. The earth's population is constantly exposed to natural background radiation from the strata making up the surface of the planet and from cosmic radiation, to which strictly controlled man-made quantities are added from power generation, medical applications, materials quality control, luminous surface treatments, forensic science and a range of industrial operations, together with fall-out from weapons testing.

Concentrations and received doses of radioactivity can be measured at very low levels with comparative ease.

The Becquerel (Bq) is a unit of activity equal to one nuclear disintegration per second and has replaced the Curie (Ci) which was based on the activity of one gram of radium $(3.7 \times 10^{10}$ Bq = 1 Ci). The absorbed radiation dose is measured in terms of the Gray (Gy), defined as the receipt of 1 Joule per Kg of material exposed, which replaces the rad or *r*adiation *a*bsorbed *d*ose, (1 Gy = 100 rads). As the type of radiation is an important characteristic in its potential for damage to health, fast neutrons being, for instance, ten times more harmful than a comparable dose of X-rays, a compensating biological factor has to be introduced into dose measurements, the unit of dose equivalence being the Sievert (Sv), i.e.

$$\text{Dose equivalent} = \text{absorbed dose} \times \text{quality factor (Sv = Gy} \times \text{QF)}$$

In the U.K. background radiation is responsible for some 70% of the total annual dose absorbed by the public, being on average about 1000 μSv per annum, with a range from 750 μSv per annum in South-east England to 1150 μSv per annum in North-east Scotland. World-wide, the range may extend to 3000 μSv per annum, with a few areas as high as 10 000 μSv per annum. The dose received from medical applications varies widely according to whether or not an individual undergoes any diagnostic or treatment procedures in any year, but, as a broad average, totals about 450 μSv per annum. Other man-made exposures, including weapons testing fall-out, account for a further 15—20 μSv per annum. It is evident that even one diagnostic X-ray or a change in the area of residence may result in a much larger increment to an individual's annual received dose than the normal effects of all industrial and military operations.

The International Commission for Radiological Protection (ICRP) is an authorative body composed mainly of medical personnel, without representatives of the nuclear industry, which makes recommendations having a strong persuasive influence on national governments in the control of ionizing radiations. The Commission's view is that exposure to radiation should only be permitted where a net positive benefit accrues and should be as low as can reasonably be achieved, and, in any case, within prescribed recommended dose limits, the limit for exposure of the public being a total of 5000 μSv per annum (whole body, blood forming organs and gonads).

Chemical energy in fuel is released during combustion by the rearrangement of forces holding the component parts of atoms together. Much greater energy is made available in thermal nuclear reactors by bombardment of the nuclei of Uranium-235 atoms with neutrons. The breaking of the forces binding the nuclear particles together not only brings about the release of energy, mainly in the form of heat, but causes the emission of neutrons which promote further fissions and the maintenance of a chain reaction, provided a critical mass of the fuel is assembled. The reaction is controlled by neutron-absorbing boron rods lowered into the core and a moderator of graphite or water, to slow the speed of the neutrons which would otherwise pass through the fuel atoms without splitting them. The heat produced is conveyed through the medium of carbon dioxide gas or water to be used for the generation of steam for electricity production in the same way as that from combustion processes. A thick concrete biological shield encloses the reactor.

In fast reactors, the speed of the neutrons is not slowed and the core contains a relatively small and concentrated quantity of plutonium, obtainable by separation from the spent fuel removed from thermal reactors, where it has been produced in low concentrations as a result of the fission of uranium. The fast reactor can be operated as a consumer of plutonium, or, by surrounding the core with a blanket of non-fissionable Uranium-238, as a breeder of plutonium, using the abundant neutrons emitted from the edge of the core to convert U-238 into Pu-239 over a period of years. Uranium-238, being the predominant isotope present in naturally-occurring uranium (99.3%) also forms the major component of spent thermal reactor fuel, and its use in this way enables much more complete extraction of the energy content of the original fuel to be achieved. The very high heat output of fast reactors necessitates a two-stage system of heat transfer, molten sodium being used as the primary coolant and a second-stage heat exchanger transferring the energy to water for steam generation.

In Britain, site licencing of nuclear installations is in the hands of the Health and Safety Executive whilst the discharge of materials to the environment is controlled by the Department of the Environment (or Welsh/Scottish Offices, as appropriate) and the Ministry of Agriculture, Fisheries and Food. Transport of radioactive substances is under the surveillance of the Departments of Transport and Trade. All these bodies operate within a legislative framework based on ICRP basic standards, supplemented by the research of the Department of Health and Social Security, and the Medical Research Council and the advice of the National Radiological Protection Board. The regulatory system is designed to ensure the independence of the production and control aspects of the nuclear power industry, without, of course, absolving the producers from their own safety responsibilities.

Safety analysis is concerned with the relative probability of the occurrence of natural and man-made disasters and the severity of their effects. Quite common events may be accepted as part of the risk of everyday living. For instance, the Building Research Establishment (1981) has noted newspaper reports of 95 deaths and 150 serious injuries resulting from gales in the period 1962–80, yet there has been no widespread alarm. The less common and more serious phenomena of hurricanes and earthquakes, although inflicting injury and death on only a tiny percentage of the earth's population in any year, are nevertheless fairly frequent as news items affecting some part of the globe, yet people have not seen fit to evacuate regions subject to these natural disasters. Voluntarily accepted hazards, such as private aviation, cigarette smoking and dangerous sports present risks which would not be tolerated from industry and public utilities. Nuclear operations must reach safety standards sufficient to reduce risks to levels readily accepted from the more remote natural disasters.

Reactor safety must be constantly directed towards preventing the release of fission products into the environment as the result of an accident. It is a factor which is comprehensively involved in the design, construction and operation of installations.

The basis of safety at the design stage is the estimation of all the possible modes of failure and the incorporation of measures, duplicated and triplicated where necessary, to counter them. The concept of 'maximum credible accident', which must be accommodated without significant danger to the public, takes into account the fact that the art of prediction is not always perfect and that occasionally, at very long intervals, unpredictable events do happen. Whilst this does not provide a guarantee of absolute safety, it is designed to ensure that the residual risk is so small as to be far outweighed by the benefits of the use of nuclear power. Construction for safety demands the highest quality of materials, work and supervision backed up by testing at all stages of assembly. Operational safety depends on the provision of systems which fail-safe and automatically prevent manual over-riding into unsafe conditions. This must be supported by a painstaking programme of inspection and maintenance.

It was the view of the Royal Commission on Environmental Pollution (sixth report, 1976) that the hazards posed by reactor accidents did not warrant the abandonment of nuclear power for that reason alone, although the risks should be taken into account in decisions on future development.

There is a strong input of social as well as scientific opinion when the issues raised by nuclear power are examined. The great increase in efficiency promised by plutonium-fuelled reactors is likely to lead to pressure for their adoption on economic grounds. If growth in the production and use of plutonium is permitted, opportunities for theft and diversion for use in terrorist weapons will present a threat requiring the most serious counter-measures. A wide range of opinion will need to be studied when assessing the acceptability of the security arrangements necessary to safeguard such a potentially dangerous commodity.

The transport of spent nuclear fuels has been the subject of concern because of the significantly hazardous nature of some of the by-products. The toxicity of Uranium fuel is little greater than that of many other substances in common industrial use and it is not a particularly high radiation hazard. Fuel elements become hazardous after irradiation in a reactor because of the transformation of some of the Uranium into Caesium-137, Strontium-90 and the group of long-lived nuclides, termed actinides, which includes Plutonium-239. Elaborate precautions are necessary to protect the cans containing these highly radioactive substances. They are removed to disposal sites in flasks of immense bulk, strength and shielding capacity, segregated from other cargoes, particularly explosives, which might have an effect on the integrity of the flask in the event of an accident. It is further necessary to divide and contain loads so that there is no possibility of a critical mass of fissile material being assembled as the result of a collision. The flasks are monitored by external radiological surveys before dispatch and after removal of the contents at the point of disposal before they are returned empty. Contingency plans have been formulated to take account of the possible types of accident which might occur to these cargoes and emergency teams are readily available to monitor and control any incident. Since the rail transport of irradiated nuclear fuels began in Britain in 1962, there has not been any incident involving the damage of flasks and the release of radioactive substances.

The disposal of radioactive waste is a matter requiring the most meticulous care in view of its hazardous nature and the extremely long half-lives of some of the radionuclides involved. Half-life ($T\frac{1}{2}$) is defined by reference to the negative exponential decrease in the activity of a substance over a period (Fig. 9.5), the interval at which it occurs being specific to the isotope and element concerned and ranging from less than 1×10^{-6} seconds to more than 1×10^{6} years.

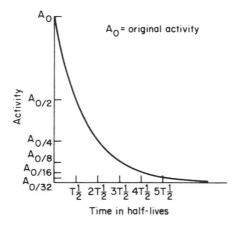

Fig. 9.5   Decay of radioactivity with time.

The basic options for waste disposal are concerned with preventing the return of releases to the ecosystem or humans by (*i*) controlled dispersal and (*ii*) containment during decay. Irradiation of waste to reduce actinide concentration has been proposed and, if ultimately found feasible, would be an attractive proposition, reducing the problem to that of dealing with relatively short-lived radioactive sub-stances, rather than those with half-lives measured in thousands of years. This process might take place at the expense of increased production of low level waste and its development to a practical level would be time-consuming and expensive. The more remote possibilities of removal to space and disposal under the polar ice-caps do not offer safe and serious options for consideration at the present time.

Controlled dispersal to the atmosphere and sea already takes place with low activity wastes, subject to international agreements. About half of the British releases arise from power generation, the remainder from radiotherapy and industry. The justification for this practice is reliance on swift dilution of the waste to levels well within ICRP safety limits for the public, and is thus similar to many other instances of disposal of hazardous materials. At present, nuclear wastes are pro-duced only by a relatively small number of agencies, world-wide, so their amounts, locations and methods of control are a matter of reasonably easy surveillance. As the use of nuclear energy spreads, increasing attention will have to be paid to waste disposal to ensure that uniform standards of safety are applied throughout the world. More so perhaps than with any other pollutant of the environment, the room for mistakes here is minimal.

In the U.K. some 1000 m^3 of medium and high activity liquid is contained in double-walled stainless steel tanks enclosed by concrete. The high heat output necessitates constant agitation of the liquid and cooling by water circulation. Naturally, the system requires continuous monitoring for leakage. The inconvenience of these procedures and the projected growth in volume of accumulated wastes to 1800–2700 m^3 by the year 2000 has prompted the search for a system of solidifi-cation which would permit storage with less supervision and a further reduction of the risk of leakage, with the ultimate objective of permitting permanent disposal in situations not subject to natural or man-made disturbance.

The feasibility of encapsulating high-level wastes in stable glasses which would remain non-reactive under the demanding conditions of heat and radiation in deep underground storage places has been established in principle. These blocks would require metal cladding as a further protection against hostile physical environments. Permanent disposal requires sites free from the risk of corrosion and leaching of the contents and disruption by natural events such as meteorite impact or volcanic disturbance, and the effects of possible future ground erosion and glaciation. Although the development of vitrification technology is well advanced, the U.K. government decided in December 1982 not to proceed with plans to investigate possible underground storage sites, but the option for reconsideration remains open.

As supplies of fossil fuels inevitably decline, more and more nations will be forced towards a choice of whether to take the nuclear energy path. Risks must be seen in the context of energy production by other means, particularly the emission of gaseous and particulate pollution by more traditional methods of power genera-tion and the environmental consequences of the disposal of solid waste from coal-fired stations. With care, a standard of safety acceptable to the majority of the population, at least in politically and socially stable communities, can be attained.

Britain's hospitals are crowded with victims of the use of tobacco and the abuse of motor vehicles, the latter being responsible for almost 7000 deaths in 1973, an annual risk of about 1 in 7000. No such allegations can be made against the nuclear industry. The verdict on its future development must be reached by balancing the risks, problems and social implications of using nuclear power against those of seeking alternative energy sources and the risks which would undoubtedly result from a world shortage of energy.

10
Aspects of the social environment

The environment in which the greatest part of our lives is spent is the home and from the earliest times humans have devoted considerable energy towards providing themselves with a secure and comfortable dwelling. The success of their efforts has naturally always been influenced by the prevailing social and economic conditions.

10.1 Housing — physical factors

The evils of disrepair, dampness, poor lighting, inadequate sanitation, bad arrangement and overcrowding arising from low quality urban development have, since the 1800s, been the subject of public concern and varying degrees of action. In recent years the problems of the lack of physical and environmental amenity and the stresses of multiple occupation have been recognized and a newer and previously unsuspected correlation between poor health and certain types of modern housing is now claiming attention. It has been reported, for instance, that children under the age of ten living in multi-storey flats may experience up to twice the incidence of upper respiratory infection found in house dwellers (Hird, 1966).

The link between low-quality housing and poor physical health has not always been easy to prove and many studies, whilst purporting to show a cause-effect relationship, have failed to allow for the numerous other social and economic effects which influence health. In any community, it is likely that the occupants of the worst quality housing will also be at a disadvantage in respect of their nutrition, clothing, medical care and education. They will also occupy a low relative position in the economic order which compels them to be employed in the more hazardous and unhealthy types of occupation. Accepting a definition of health which stretches beyond the absence of physical disease leads readily to the association of housing with well-being and compels the conclusion that housing must be regarded as a significant factor in the total environment.

10.1.1 Historical aspects

In developed countries, the turning point in housing history has usually coincided with industrialization as rural populations have poured into rapidly expanding towns to occupy cheap, crowded dwellings hastily erected at a high density. In the British experience, this urbanization was at its peak during the period 1790—1830 and was accompanied by a 50% population increase. Houses were built to provide local pools of labour for expanding industry and costs involved in the quality of materials, methods of construction and provision of facilities were kept to an absolute minimum. In these conditions, water-borne and infectious diseases spread rapidly and infestations were virtually uncontrolled. Attempts were made to rectify matters by an abundance of legislation in the Victorian era directed towards the improvement of building control, town planning and the provision of better housing with such improved sanitary arrangements as were being developed at the time.

The physical environment of mass-produced housing of the 1800s was created with little regard for the principles of building hygiene. Streets and courts were arranged for maximum dwelling density; orientation, privacy and open space around buildings were not considered to be important factors. Houses were entered from narrow streets, usually without the benefit of even small areas of private space at the front. Some of the worst of Britain's slums were constructed on the 'back-to-back' principle, with other buildings abutting the rear as well as both sides of the houses, sacrificing any effective ventilation of the ground floor rear rooms to meet the objective of maximum land use. On sloping ground, the construction of basement rooms was difficult to avoid and many almost toally underground rooms were to be found in hilly towns. In later conventional terraced housing, kitchen facilities were usually provided in an annexe structure at the rear, which occupied a substantial slice of the rear 'garden' and often contributed to serious overshadowing. In the more spacious of these houses, the rear annexe might extend to two stories, a small bedroom being formed on the upper floor. Because of restricted space and the pressures for economy of construction this room would usually be entered directly from the main rear bedroom.

Cheapness of construction was assisted by the use of inferior materials, good quality local stone often being rejected in favour of cheaper, poorly-fired bricks. The annexe structures were often particularly bad, being built of a single thickness of brickwork with poor resistance to penetrating dampness, on inadequate foundations with a simple flagstone floor laid directly on compacted earth. Roofs were commonly of the centre valley gutter type, again for cheapness. Dampness flourished in these houses and the inferior construction of the annexes led commonly to varying degrees of instability, sometimes causing these additions to part company from the main structure at roof level. The roof itself was not amenable to accommodating any movement of the house and was often subject to recurrent leaks when settlement took place. The entry of water caused premature decay of the general fabric of the rest of the building.

Water supplies in those days had advanced little beyond the era of the village pump and might typically be obtained from a standpipe serving a group of houses, though this arrangement was later to give way to the provision of individual supplies. Sewage disposal was equally rudimentary, in the worst cases consisting only of earth closets or primitive water-carried systems amounting to little more than the urban version of the ditch. The earlier WCs were of the hopper type, with untrapped central outlets providing free passage for rats and odours up through the system unprotected by a water seal.

In these cramped dwellings large families were born and raised in the face of severe physical difficulties. In England in 1841 expectation of life at birth was 40 years (male) and 42 years (female) and by the year 1900 these expectations had been raised only to 44 and 48 years respectively. It is a matter for speculation as to what contribution better housing conditions made to the total overall improvement in the health of the population, but by 1952, after prodigious efforts in the fields of slum clearance and house improvement, the corresponding figures were 66 and 72 years respectively.

Early legislation provided for the enactment of Building Byelaws by local authorities and from the 1870s houses were constructed to the minimum requirements of these codes, based on model standards adapted to local conditions and surviving to the present day in the form of Building Regulations, now applying uniformly throughout the country. Although the level of the standards prescribed by the early Byelaws was meagre compared with modern practice, a gradual improvement to Britain's housing stock was achieved as new dwellings built under this system of control formed an increasing part of the urban scene. Provision for the clearance of unfit houses and badly-arranged areas was also made.

By the 1930s, with the added assistance of subsidies for new building, considerable progress had been made towards replacing the worst of the industrial revolution legacy. Prior to 1939 dwelling construction was proceeding at the rate of some 300 000 units per annum, but the outbreak of hostilities in the Second World War reduced this to a total of only 200 000 built through the total six year period of the war. This was insufficient even to replace the 225 000 destroyed by enemy action. In the immediate post-war years a deficit approaching two million dwellings had been accumulated and over half a million had sustained severe damage. Faced with the pressing problem of housing those with literally no roof over their heads, little progress could be made in improving housing for the rest of the community or renewing those houses which had deteriorated from bad to unfit through unavoidable neglect during the war years. To these difficulties was added the problem of a population expansion as normal family life was resumed.

As late as 1953, 65% of the privately rented dwellings in Britain were over 65 years old, but it was not until the late 1950s that serious progress with slum clearance could be resumed. By that time, normal supplies of building materials were once more available and private house development had been able to get under way again. Prefabricated houses had mushroomed in the immediate post-war years as a solution to the urgent needs of the homeless, and their success was such that many were to outlast their original expected ten-year life by a factor of three or more. The next decade was to see vigorous (some would say ruthless) demolition of worn-out city areas as green-field sites on the fringes of urban areas were developed and in other cases complete new towns were created. In the better large scale post-war housing developments social needs were recognized and leisure and community activities were included.

A 'community' is something which is frequently spoken about, more problematic to define and extraordinarily difficult to create. Inhabitants of inner suburbs, whilst welcoming a move to vastly improved physical surroundings, often found themselves ill at ease with a changed social environment as the populations of compact, well-rooted city areas were dispersed to housing estates. The bad housing environment, for all its difficulties, often carried with it certain conveniences; familiarity with neighbours, easy access to shopping, well-established local meeting places and, perhaps, a philosophy of shared problems. It might have been expected that the population of new estates would be healthier as a result of better housing, but studies have shown higher rates of consulting medical practitioners by the people who have made these moves. Even where serious physical ailments are not present, such increases may indicate increased anxiety, a further reflection on the mental and social aspects of health.

10.1.2   Multiple occupation

Whilst for many people the transition from old, worn-out housing to a new home and style of life was taking place, other problems were emerging from a different class of old housing. Owners of large good quality property found themselves facing increasing difficulties in maintaining and heating houses which were becoming increasingly unfashionable and unmanageable in an era of compactness, convenience and smaller families. Multiple occupation was seen as a solution to the problem of generating the income to run a house which was too large and expensive for single family use. Unfortunately, although space was abundant in Victorian houses built for occupation by the prosperous sections of the community at that time, the building services and facilities were totally inadequate for several families.

In the better instances, large dwellings could be skillfully converted to provide several desirable apartments within the one structure, each with its own water supply, sanitation, heating system, cooking facilities and a satisfactory degree of privacy. In many cases, however, shared facilities ranging from barely acceptable to grossly inadequate, were provided. Fire precautions and means of escape were often non-existent. Water supply pipes were often inadequate to serve additional sinks and water closets, where these were provided. Electrical systems could well be grossly overloaded. Washing, cooking and refuse disposal facilities used in common and being no-one's specific responsibility were likely to become neglected and filthy.

The demands on the maintenance of the fabric increased with the occupancy, but were often neglected, particularly where absentee landlords saw the opportunity for the quick extraction of profit with minimum investment. A blocked drain or dangerous staircase is a serious enough problem in a one-family house, but is multiplied many times over with several families living under one roof. In certain houses in multiple occupation the most squalid and stressful conditions were allowed to develop by a totally unscrupulous section of the landlord group, whose aims were enforced by harassment, illegal evictions and intimidatory practices of every kind. In other cases, property owners were caught in a financial trap by under-financed operations and spiralling overhead costs which frustrated their genuine wish to provide accommodation of a high standard.

Legislative controls helped in the alleviation of the worst of these problems, but were constrained by the size of the problem and enforcement difficulties. Fiscal policy was used to support penal legislation and extensive use has been made of improvement grants to encourage the division of large houses into apartments, as well as the modernization of individual homes needing the provision of basic facilities. The grant system has recently been extended to encompass certain major structural repair works.

10.1.3   Contemporary problems

National House Condition Surveys conducted by the Department of the Environment in England showed that the number of unfit dwellings remained relatively constant at 1.1 to 1.2 million over the years 1971—81, and tended to be scattered throughout the housing stock rather than concentrated in areas requiring comprehensive clearance and redevelopment. An encouraging reduction in the number of dwellings lacking the basic amenities of an indoor WC, bathroom, washbasin, sink and hot water supply was also noted (1971, 16%; 1981, 5%) and there were indications that the remaining 0.9 million unimproved houses were in that condition mainly because of considerations such as the occupant's age or the inconvenience of having works carried out, rather than financial problems alone. Dwellings in need of major repair (works in excess of £7000 at 1981 prices) had increased over the ten-year period and suggest that a serious cause of future housing problems may be under-financed owner-occupation, particularly amongst the young with incomes heavily committed to mortgage repayments and retired people whose resources have been severely eroded by inflation.

The worst physical housing conditions, which can only be dealt with by demolition or extensive reconstruction, are expected to be in evidence only in worn-out buildings. Nevertheless, there are examples of avoidable defects to be seen in new dwellings. Unsatisfactory detail design and the poor application of new construction methods, together with inferior materials and workmanship have, not infrequently, led to the early deterioration of the fabric or its components and the entry of the elements. Noise transmission has been found to be a widespread problem where careless construction of party walls has greatly reduced their theoretical sound insulating properties. Extensive structural strengthening has been necessary in a number of multi-storey buildings in which high-alumina cement had been used, because of the risk of premature deterioration of concrete structural members fabricated from this material.

Some modern building techniques and designs have brought about a considerable increase in the incidence of condensation problems. Condensation is linked to a number of factors which often interact, including the incorporation in dwellings of building materials with poor thermal insulating properties and unsatisfactory internal arrangement, particularly in flats, causing moisture-laden air from bathrooms and kitchens to be contained and cooled to condense on cold surfaces. These problems are accentuated by the trend away from open fireplaces to paraffin stoves and other forms of heating which raise humidities to problematical levels within the rooms in which they are used.

10.2 Housing — social factors

An increasing body of opinion suggests that the major problems of new housing are as much social as physical in nature. It has been sadly apparent that certain developments of well built and equipped dwellings have, through the effects of abuse and neglect, rapidly deteriorated into modern slums. The reasons for this are, no doubt, subtle and complex.

10.2.1 Housing design

Multi-storey development has featured consistently in criticism of modern housing. It is not, of course, an inherently inferior type of housing and many buildings of this kind are occupied by perfectly satisfied tenants. Although the British appear generally to adapt to flat-dwelling with less enthusiasm than other European nations, there are advantages of convenience which have an undoubted appeal for a minority. It is in the case of families with young children that the most common and valid areas of criticism arise. Parents are understandably anxious at being removed from their children playing outside at ground level, but the alternative of keeping active youngsters indoors is equally stressful. The needs of very young children are met much more satisfactorily by having access to private gardens, even if these are very small, immediately adjoining their homes and this is now recognized in the policies of many housing authorities who accept the need for every family home to possess a zone of outdoor space under the exclusive control of its occupants.

Further anxieties are occasioned by the fear of children falling from high windows and balconies, but where these are designed for increased safety by raising the sill height, they provoke objections from the older generation who experience isolation through being restricted to a very limited view of the outside world whilst seated. The disablement of lifts as a result of vandalism, poor maintenance or power cuts can be a serious problem for elderly or infirm occupants and some are poorly proportioned for the removal of stretcher cases or the dignified transport of coffins.

10.2.2   Estate planning

The experience of grossly overcrowded inner-city areas of the past induced a reaction whereby low-rise, low-density developments were created in outlying areas to rehouse the populations of the urban slums. As pressure on scarce resources of land became severe, a logical solution appeared to be the increase of residential density by building skywards. Tall buildings, however, require space around them to prevent overshadowing and, in view of the objections against high-rise developments, modern policies seek the achievement of high population densities in updated versions of traditional low-rise housing. Many successful schemes prove that it is possible, by careful design and planning of the whole site area, to maximize land use while still preserving familiar dwelling types.

The traditional house and garden provides opportunities for informal and uncommitted social contact — the talk over the garden fence, the spontaneous and casual invitation to coffee — which are severely limited in the encapsulated world of high-rise flats, where such approaches must be more planned and positive. The communal areas of such buildings are a 'no man's land' where the presence of strangers may be suspected but insufficient reason in itself for challenge. Door-to-door callers, however legitimate their business, are liable to find a distinct atmosphere of insularity, unless known personally to the occupants. Residents are likely to be less willing to participate in social or market surveys than their counterparts in conventional houses. Despite this insularity, noise from neighbours on all sides, above and below, may seriously interfere with privacy.

The answer to the avoidance of problems in housing is not completely known, and much will depend on the background and social mix of the occupants of any development. Experience suggests that detailed architectural design plays an important part. Popular and respected housing schemes provide privacy and a sense of security in the dwelling types and layout. Homes are preferably entered by a private door at ground level, approached by a path which takes a natural course, rather than a route which is more appealing on the drawing board than in practice. It is interesting to see the well-worn paths, beaten across open grassed areas, on many housing estates, neatly by-passing the paved access provided. Grouped car parking, screened from direct view and often situated some distance from the dwelling, is superficially attractive but not generally liked by vehicle owners, who prefer simple and convenient arrangements whereby they can exercise some supervision over their possessions.

The poor definition of private and public areas of space is a source of conflict between older residents and the younger generation who rarely select their meeting places and play areas with any awareness of the annoyance which their gatherings, however innocent in purpose, can cause. Land not specifically enclosed for any purpose can quickly become a harbouring place for litter and may, in the absence of regular maintenance, deteriorate into a rubbish dump. Economies in grass cutting and the general care of communal areas contribute to an overall run-down appearance. Residents do not generally share the enthusiasm shown by some architects for the extensive provision of communal, rather than private, leisure and recreation space.

It is for these and associated reasons that some estates are successful and others give the impression of a 'human warehouse' environment from the time of first occupation, with their confusion of pathways, decked access to upper-storey entrances and a general atmosphere of the rabbit-warren, however luxurious and well-equipped the individual portions of the scheme may be. Further scope exists for social studies to determine what contribution these factors make to juvenile crime, marital strife, child abuse, vandalism and the other symptoms of problem housing areas.

10.3   Leisure and health

The contribution of leisure pursuits to environmental problems is not insignificant. The personal accident hazards involved in competitive sports, climbing, caving and a variety of activities are, of course, fairly evident, but a range of more insidious effects of noise and pollution also exist. These require recognition and avoidance, or, at least, mitigation.

10.3.1   Noise

Pollution and noise from traffic have been previously considered (Chaps 8 and 9) and, in the context of leisure activities, it may be relevant to enquire what proportion of the total problem is attributable to journeys made for recreational rather than commercial purposes. Holiday traffic has been such a serious cause of road congestion in popular tourist areas of Britain at peak periods that the designation of special relief routes has been necessary. The heavy goods vehicle is often blamed as the main culprit in traffic noise and on a comparison with the individual car this view is, no doubt, justified. This is not necessarily the case when it is merged with other classes of traffic. Calculations by the Transport and Road Research Laboratory (1974) examined variations in total noise emissions with different combinations of vehicle silencing, traffic flow and proportion of heavy vehicles. One calculation, assuming 10% goods vehicles in a traffic flow of 400 vehicles per hour, predicted a reduction in the L_{10} dB(A) level of 1.4 dB(A) following the silencing of lorries by an additional 10 dB(A) and 4.0 dB(A) from additional silencing of only 5 dB(A) applied to cars. The expansion of provincial airports to handle night-flights for summer holiday aircraft normally meets with considerable resistance and resentment by local residents.

The internal combustion engine is also responsible for many noise problems away from the public roads. These will be familiar to people living near the sites of organized motor sport events, who also have to contend with the congestion and pollution problems caused by the convergence of large numbers of vehicle-borne spectators to the site. To the great annoyance of local inhabitants, an increasing number of young people are taking to fields and other open spaces with small, but nevertheless noisy, motorcycles, free from the licencing and other legal controls which apply to riding on the highway. These machines are now being produced in sizes suitable for riders down to the age of four. On an even smaller scale, the tiny engines of model aircraft can be guilty of considerable disturbance in and around public recreation areas because of the wide propagation of noise from airborne sources.

Local Authorities have had to deal with a steady increase in the number of complaints about noise from entertainment places over the last decade (see Fig. 9.4). The fashion for extremely loud music in clubs and discotheques is not universally welcomed by the patrons and rarely appreciated by neighbours. Unlike many industrial noise problems, the character of which is fixed and amenable to measurement, analysis and rectification, entertainment noise fluctuates greatly in volume and frequency and is thus more difficult to characterize and control. There are substantial problems in designing acoustic insulation of buildings, since the attenuation properties of a wall increase by a theoretical maximum of only 6 dB for each doubling of either the mass of the wall or the frequency of the sound, and attentuation is severely reduced by any door or window opening. The problem is at its worst when a party wall is shared with other premises. Popular 'beat' music usually contains a loud bass group of frequencies and any attempts to reduce transmission through the wall by a worthwhile amount usually imply an impracticable increase in the thickness of the wall.

Considerable conflict occurs when noisy entertainments are newly introduced into a quiet neighbourhood, as, for instance, when the local inn sets out to attract more trade by recruiting a band or disc-jockey. The problems are increased by late-night vehicle movement, shouting and the possibilities of a variety of other high-spirited or anti-social behaviour.

Noise doses many times larger than the present permitted upper industrial limit of 90 dB(A) 8-hour Leq can be received during an evening's entertainment at a club or concert. It is possible that the risk of hearing damage in these situations has been overestimated and that relatively short and infrequent exposures may not be as damaging as a crude assessment of the measured dose would first suggest. In the present state of knowledge it is not, however, possible to predict the effects of frequent exposure over a long period and industrial experience should encourage caution. It may also be noted that indoor swimming pools can be very noisy places, when the clamour of an enthusiastic crowd is reflected around the hard, non-absorbant interior of the building.

The use of firearms in sport is a generally safe form of recreation, as the disciplinary rules of gun clubs and police control of weapons minimize the risks of injury. The risk of hearing damage, is, however, a matter of some importance. The noise from a .44 calibre pistol can easily exceed 135 dB at 1m. This approaches the upper limit of 150 dB for 'impulse' noise (i.e. noise measured with a sound level meter capable of response to a very sudden increase in level, the standard 'impulse' response time being 0.035 seconds) to which the unprotected ear should never be exposed for even the briefest period. Noise-induced hearing loss is not an uncommon condition in ex-servicemen repeatedly exposed to gunfire in earlier life and is being increasingly recognized in others as having resulted from the sporting use of firearms.

Levels of airborne lead in indoor firing ranges have been studied in the U.S.A.

and Britain. Investigations by the Avon, Gloucestershire and Somerset Environment Monitoring Committee (1979) representing local authorities in the west of England, revealed airborne lead levels between 36.2 μg m^{-3} and 4700 μg m^{-3} under varying conditions of weapon, ammunition and range use. Of 30 results in the study, 27 exceeded the recommended maximum time-weighted average industrial exposure (TLV — TWA) of 150 μg m^{-3}. Very few people are exposed to indoor shooting range conditions for extended periods and it is unlikely that all the airborne lead is present as particles of respirable size, but this is another source of potential lead hazard to which users should be alerted. This is even more important if, as is quite commonly the case, food or drink is likely to be consumed in the premises. One of the ranges surveyed was also used at other times as a skittle alley and venue for social events.

10.3.2 Water sports and activities

New patterns of leisure activities on and in water have implications for public health and the environment. Power boat racing on inland stretches of water has been received enthusiastically by the public and commercial sponsorship of competitive events has ensured that they are widely publicized and supported. There is an area of obvious potential conflict between these activities and the interests of nearby residents, having regard to noise emissions and the congregation of spectators. Some control of individual craft is exercised by the regulations of the Union Internationale Motonautique, which specify a noise limit of 85 dB (with a 10 dB tolerance) measured at 25 m from the front, rear and sides of the competing craft 1.25 m above the water surface. In the U.K., a draft Code of Practice is at present under discussion to make further provision for protection against the intrusion of noise. The deciding factors in the acceptability of this sport appear to be frequency and duration of events. Even where the noise levels are high, few but the most sensitive have serious objections to an annual event of a few days' duration, but complaints increase and gain justification with more frequent occurrences.

The dangers of swimming in grossly polluted water are well-recognized and the physical properties of such water are usually unpleasant enough to be a strong deterrent to entry. Moderate pollution may not be so easily detected, but may give rise to the presence of pathogens. Although typhoid and paratyphoid fevers, dysentery and gastroenteritis are usually transmitted by food, they are quite capable of being contracted through swimming in contaminated river, canal and estuarial waters and leptospirosis is a recognized risk. Diving, water-skiing and boating may take place at venues rejected for straightforward swimming but, of course, still involve varying degrees of risk of immersion in the water and contact with any pathogens present.

10.3.3 Swimming bath management

Swimming bath management is very much concerned with water cleanliness and treatment for the protection of users against infectious diseases. Filtration of water during circulation is essential to remove the debris of hair, skin cells, bodily secretions and dirt introduced by each entrant to the pool. Chlorination is applied to control microorganisms. The practice of chlorination was in use long before a complete understanding of the complex chemical processes involved had been gained. Gaseous chlorine is immediately taken up in the oxidation of organic matter and the dosage must be sufficient to provide free, available chlorine to perform its continually changing conditions of load. Over-chlorinated water can be treated with potassium permanganate or sodium thiosulphate to adjust the residual level.

The eyes are susceptible to both chemical and microbiological hazards when exposed to swimming bath waters. They are constantly bathed in a complex fluid with a pH of approximately 7.4 and exposure to chlorine in high concentrations or over extended periods may alter this value and produce irritation, blurred vision, lachrymation (tears) and other visual disturbances. Conjunctivitis is a relatively minor risk in the water and exposure to the variety of organisms which can cause this condition is more likely to be encountered in the shared use of towels. The expulsion of mucus from the nose and throat is not uncommon during swimming, especially when diving, and being resistant to the penetration of disinfectants, may carry ear infections to other swimmers, gaining access through the outer ear and being forced through the eustachian tube by pressure changes whilst the ear is under water.

The risk of contacting gastro-intestinal diseases is rare in properly run pools and the fears of the spread of poliomyelitis through public bathing, commonly expressed in the 1950s when this disease was prevalent in a population then largely unvaccinated, would probably have been better directed towards poor hygiene and person-to-person contacts in changing rooms and sanitary conveniences, rather than the pool water. Nevertheless, there are other conditions which are specifically associated with the use of swimming baths.

The fungal infection 'athlete's foot' and plantar warts, caused by a virus, can reach epidemic proportions in populations using poorly designed and managed pools. These infections, which in some stages are difficult to detect by inspection, are harboured in worn and pitted floors, particularly if any wood is contained in the structure. They are controllable, if not completely preventable, by frequent attention to the cleaning and maintenance of floor surfaces. The provision of disinfectant foot-baths, sited between the changing rooms and the pool in such a position that their use is not easily avoided, are of some assistance. Other skin diseases are associated with pools — the organism *Pseudomonas aeruginosa*, which causes a rash, is a potential problem in therapeutic pools, where the higher temperatures favour bacterial multiplication if chlorination is ineffective. 'Swimming pool granuloma', a persistent disease causing ulceration, attributed to *Mycobacterium marinum*, an organism producing a condition similar to tuberculosis in fish, can be contracted through skin abrasions, but is, again, uncommon in adequately chlorinated waters.

The rare, but frequently fatal, condition of primary amoebic meningoencephalitis has been recognized in recent years. It is believed to be contracted through the mucous membranes of the nose. The infection may be present in warm waters contaminated by soil and can be harboured in dirt in cracks and crevices in the pool structure, but is unlikely to survive for long in adequately chlorinated water.

11
The working environment

Fully-employed adults spend up to 25% of their life actually at work, and further time in preparation and travelling. The obvious necessity to obtain subsistence is the prime motivator behind this daily routine, but very much more should be involved — the sense of achievement, identification with a group and the fulfilment of ambition. Despite frequent complaints about the daily routine of labour, unemployment is recognized as degrading, demoralizing, damaging to psychological and perhaps ultimately to physical health. A large number of people will undoubtedly be facing this as a long-term problem in the future. The working environment has a close association with health because its physical, chemical, biological and social hazards can have serious effects on the human being.

11.1 Physical hazards

The physical hazards of the working environment include noise, vibration, heat, cold, radiation and extreme variations in atmospheric pressure.

11.1.1 Noise

The noise generated by heavy engineering equipment, internal combustion engines, pneumatic drills and a multitude of other mechanical sources, in addition to the problems of fatigue, inconvenience and inefficiency may be positively injurious to the function of hearing by causing damage to the delicate mechanisms of the ear. The first signs of noise-induced hearing loss in more susceptible individuals may be detected after extended exposure to noise in excess of 80 db(A). The incidence of this industrial disability has long been noted in the shipbuilding and weaving industries and over the years it has been recorded in a wide range of occupations.

Short-term exposure to high noise levels causes fatigue to the hearing (temporary threshold shift) which normally corrects itself, except in the case of grossly high intensities, after a period of time spent away from the source. With repeated and extended exposure, the damage gradually becomes irrepairable and the victim is aware of the onset of disability. The frequency content of the consonants in speech is higher than that of vowel sounds and the first symptom is likely to be confusion between spoken words. Difficulties will become more serious if the condition is allowed to worsen by continuing exposure, when a gradually increasing band of frequencies will be affected. Later, when additional hearing losses through the process of ageing (presbycousis) are added, the sufferer will bear the burden of a handicap causing partial isolation in the retirement years.

Noise induced hearing loss is shown characteristically in audiometry by a significant loss of sensitivity in the region of 4 KHz with some degree of recovery in the higher frequency bands. This pattern can easily be distinguished from that of presbycousis, where, with increasing age, progressively larger losses are registered through bands of increasing frequency (Fig. 11.1).

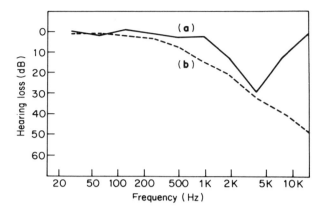

Fig. 11.1   Theoretical audiograms comparing (a) noise-induced hearing loss and (b) presbycousis.

The current U.K. maximum recommended limit for exposure to noise contained in the Department of Employment Code of Practice is 90 dB(A), averaged over an 8-hour working day. In this case, the average referred to is the Leq index, used to give appropriate weight to the logarithmically increasing amount of energy contained in noise above 90 dB(A) (see Chap. 8, p. 141). Because of individual susceptibility, even adherence to this standard gives no guarantee of protection to all workers and a number will still suffer varying degress of handicap. For this reason, the Code of Practice encourages employers to aim for lower noise exposures and many occupational hygienists would like to see a maximum Leq of 80 dB(A) enacted.

Accurate measurements can, of course, only be made with sound level meters, but suspicion of excessive levels should be aroused in any workplace where shouting is necessary to converse over the noise. In such cases a survey with instruments is warranted and the noise dose meter provides a convenient way of measuring the total received by a user during a working day. These instruments are typically pocket-sized, with a weight of 200 gm or so and a microphone extension which can be attached to the lapel or to safety headwear, so causing little incumbrance during day-long wear.

The most satisfactory ways of guarding against excessive noise exposure are the substitution of quiet machinery and the enclosure of noisy processes (see p. 142). Where these methods are not practicable, protection of the individual is needed and the choice of method will depend on the characteristics of the sound, particularly its frequency spectrum. Ear muffs, mouldable plugs and glass down are all effective in varying situations. Cotton wool is of negligible value. Unfortunately all these types of personal protection cause some discomfort to the user, particularly in warm working conditions, and may induce a feeling of isolation. There are associated problems of hygiene and correct fitting and these devices must be considered second best to silencing at source.

Although noise has for some time been recognized as a problem in factories, its significance for the white collar worker has been made apparent with the arrival of computers, word processors and the use of remote terminals. In the resultant noise climate relatively simple errors have been made by programmers and sound levels in computer rooms have been found to exceed not only accepted criteria for comfortable office working conditions, but even those which would be acceptable in a workshop according to the standards adopted by some companies.

Even outside the specialized situation of the computer room, some offices are subject to noise from typing, telephones, movement and outside traffic sufficient to cause fatigue and interfere with verbal communications. The Speech Interference Level (SIL), which is calculated by taking the arithmetic average of the sound pressure levels in each of the three octave bands centred on 500, 1000 and 2000 Hz, provides a useful basis for defining ease of verbal communication. At a distance of 1 m, normal speech is likely to be intelligible when the background noise level is 58 to 60 dB, but at 4m the same ease of communication can only be achieved with a background of 46 to 48 dB. Shouted messages become difficult to hear at 4m when the ambient noise level is 65 dB, or at 2m in a climate of 77 dB. The application of this concept suggests progressively more stringent criteria being appropriate for situations where the quantity and quality of verbal communication is increasingly important. Typing pools may well be satisfactory with a SIL of 60 dB, but 45 dB is preferable for a private office, with 35 dB for conference rooms and 30 dB for live theatres and school rooms.

11.1.2 Vibration

Vibration, like noise with which it is often closely associated, can cause effects ranging from discomfort to definite physical damage, which will vary according to the frequency and amplitude of the vibration and the length of exposure. Whole-body effects are experienced most acutely at frequencies below about 30 Hz and are a potential hazard to anyone in direct physical contact with vibrating surfaces or enclosures, such as drivers of heavy machines. Any worker employed in the immediate vicinity of machinery where heavy revolving shafts or reciprocating parts are in operation may be at risk, particularly if the working platform is directly connected to the machine. The tolerance of the human body to low-frequency vibrations is much lower where the forces act in a horizontal plane, rather than on the foot-head axis.

Raynaud's Phenomenon is a condition, usually affecting the hands, arising from localized vibration. In its early stages it is characterized by whiteness of the fingers, due to damage to the blood vessels and nerves, hence its common description of 'white-finger'. Sensation is dulled and control of movement may be affected, with some pain experienced when blood circulation is restored. With minor, infrequent exposure the condition may correct itself spontaneously without lasting ill-effect, but, once established, may worsen even without further contact with vibration. The effects will be amplified as a consequence of further exposure and future attacks may be brought on by a variety of activities, particularly if the hands are exposed to cold and wet, quite unconnected with vibration. A proportion of the general population, without any history of exposure to vibration, is susceptible to similar symptoms.

Criteria of acceptability for whole-body vibration are contained in British Standard 6472 : 1984 and are designed to take into account the protection of be set which take into account the protection of comfort and the prevention of fatigue as well as the preservation of health. It is to be hoped that similar criteria will in due course be established for limiting exposure of the hands but until then, exposure to vibration should be treated cautiously. Contact time should be minimized and tasks changed periodically to give rest intervals between exposures. The source of vibration should be controlled to produce the lowest levels possible and insulation should be incorporated in the design of vibrating hand tools. Gloves help to damp vibration at the higher frequencies and have the extra advantage of protecting against cold in outside conditions, which could itself bring on an attack of Raynaud's Phenomenon in a susceptible person.

11.1.3   Temperature

The correlation between temperature and comfort needs little explanation, but the more extreme variations in temperature may lead to definite risks to the health of those exposed. The danger of heat exposure is likely to affect metallurgical process workers, miners and all who are employed in the close vicinity of sizeable furnaces.

The body takes some four to six days to acclimatize to hot conditions, the process being completed more satisfactorily with younger persons. Such adaptation rapidly disappears when the individual is removed from hot conditions and usually goes completely in three weeks. No precise temperatures can be defined to limit the effect of heat, as much depends on individual susceptibility, the degree of physical effort involved in work and protective clothing worn. Early symptoms of heat exhaustion are dizziness and nausea, often accompanied by rapid, shallow breathing and clamminess of the skin, which may even produce a cold sensation. Recovery is rapid on removal to cooler conditions, but more serious effects may ensue from prolonged exposure when excessive fluid and salt is lost from the body and a long period of rest is necessary to make good the losses. Under extreme conditions, the temperature regulation of the body can be completely disturbed and overheating progresses without control. The condition can ultimately prove fatal unless artificial external cooling is applied.

When the body temperature is lowered by exposure to severe weather conditions, such as may be found on construction works or trawlers or in cold stores, irrational behaviour may be induced, followed by unconsciousness and eventual loss of life when the temperature of the body falls to about 28°C. Local frostbite may occur even when these whole-body effects do not develop, as blood circulation is reduced to conserve heat. Air movement is a critical factor in the effects of cold and the actual temperature may effectively be lowered by many degrees by the presence of rapidly moving airstreams, such as are found near air intakes in mine ventilation systems.

11.1.4   Radiation

All forms of electro-magnetic radiation, even visible light, are potentially dangerous if the intensity is too high. Ultraviolet light, the component of sunlight which causes tanning of the skin is a familiar cause of burns (sunburn). Its effect may be made worse by simultaneous exposure to fumes of pitch and tar. Exposure to ultraviolet light is also believed to play a part in the causation of melanoma, a type of skin cancer which is more common in fair-skinned persons who live in countries where the sunshine is particularly strong and in those who spend a great deal of their time working outside. The eye is very sensitive to ultraviolet radiation and the very painful condition of 'arc eye' is a recognized hazard of the exposure of the eye to welding operations. Despite the intense discomfort of this condition it is fortunately not believed to cause any long-term damage. Other hazards of ultra-violet radiation are the production of ozone, nitrogen dioxide and phosgene in the atmosphere. The sources, apart from sunlight, are welding arcs, arc lamps, mercury vapour lamps, sterilizers and photocopiers. Control is exercised by the screening of these sources and eye and skin protection. Ultraviolet light is also an important factor in the causation of photochemical smog in the particular climatic conditions of some cities, for example, Los Angeles and Tokyo (see Chap. 8).

Infra-red radiation is a common industrial hazard, being emitted by any red-hot material, so is frequently associated with furnace operations and welding. The radiation causes skin burns similar to various stages of sunburn and, after very long exposure, cataracts in the lenses of the eyes. Screening and protection of the skin are therefore important, also the use of tinted lenses, for example, when viewing furnace operations.

Laser beams are now in common use for setting out construction works where accurate alignment of structures over considerable distances is necessary. They are amplified light beams produced in many frequencies, from ultraviolet to infra-red and not all are visible. Laser beams vary in hazard according to frequency and power and the effects may range from virtually harmless to severe destruction of tissue, especially the retina of the eye. Protection consists of the selection of the safest instruments, the separation of the beam and personnel by barriers and ade-quate warning signs. Instruments need to be properly fixed so that they will not be displaced from the target and reflective surfaces near the target should be elimin-ated. Eye protection specifically designed to guard against the effects of laser beams is available and should be widely used since, in the present state of knowledge, all laser beams should be regarded as unsafe for unprotected viewing.

Microwaves are increasingly being used around airfields in association with radar and other communications equipment and in the catering industry as the use of microwave ovens becomes more popular. Mircowaves range in length from about 1 mm to 1 m or a frequency of 300 MHz to 300 GHz. They share a number of the properties of light in that they travel in straight lines and may be reflected or trans-mitted as, for example, by metal or glass respectively, or absorbed. Particularly at the lower frequencies involved, the deep tissues of the body absorb a considerable amount of the incident energy as heat and as there is no rise in skin temperature to warn of the internal heating, these frequencies can pose a serious risk. An import-ant factor in the dispersal of internally produced heat is the vascularization of the irradiated organ, since the circulation of the blood helps greatly in heat dissipation and it is believed that lack of this physiological property in the lens of the eye accounts for the risk of cataracts developing from microwave radiation exposure. The reproductive organs are at considerable risk from high intensities at very close ranges. Changes in the central and peripheral nervous systems have been observed as a result of microwave irradiation and alterations in the thresholds for some sense organs are suspected. Some workers have reported changes in electroencephalogram patterns which may also be attributable to this source. Symptoms or associated behavioural disturbances which have been reported include pains in the eye, frontal headaches, sensations of buzzing, vibrations or pulsations, fatigue, drowsiness, irritability, depression and loss of appetite, but there is still some dispute about whether these effects are in fact due to microwave radiation. Protection of exposed individuals is difficult and is best achieved by limiting the numbers of people exposed and defining risk zones of radiation after measurement. In the United Kingdom ovens are required to comply with a Code of Practice limiting leakage to 5 mW cm^{-2} measured at 50 mm and occupational exposure is limited to 10 mW cm^{-2}. Differing opinions on acceptable levels have been stated in other countries and complete international agreement seems some way off.

Ionizing radiation is particularly insidious in its effects which range from burns, dermatitis and cateracts to cancers, particularly leukaemia, and damage to the reproductive cells causing sterility, infertility and congenital abnormalities in later generations. Alpha radiation is given off by some radioactive substances but has little range or penetrating power. This type of radiation produces intense ionization over very short distances — measured in millimetres. Externally it is thus a minimal hazard in view of its poor penetration, but it is potentially very dangerous if ingested, since it may then directly affect cellular components of vital bodily organs or systems and cause a range of effects. These are potentially serious if the dosage is excessive. Beta particles, consisting of streams of fast moving electrons, are more penetrating, but mainly affect the skin and subcutaneous tissue. The high energy X-ray and gamma radiation are extremely penetrating forms which can pass right through the body and cause a range of serious effects.

X-ray examinations for medical purposes are a prime source of radiation over and above the natural background radiation to which we are all exposed and contribute a substantial part of the excess radiation of the population, more important than the fall out from nuclear weapons testing or radiation derived from nuclear power stations (see Chap. 9, p. 148). In industry, radiography of structures and components presents potential risk and the exposure of medical and dental personnel using X-ray equipment also requires careful surveillance. In most countries very strict control over sources of radiation is imposed but scientific debate continues concerning effects and it is possible that there is no threshold below which the possibility of physiological damage can be excluded.

11.1.5   Atmospheric pressure

Divers and other workers in compressed air suffer a range of health hazards, including 'the bends', a painful condition caused by the liberation of nitrogen, dissolved in the blood at high pressures, but liberated, due to differential pressures, in the form of bubbles in the blood on over-rapid decompression. Nitrogen narcosis arises from the same cause, as does bone necrosis (damage to joints which can leave a disability similar to arthritis). Very deep diving can lead to high pressure neurological syndrome (HPNS) — symptoms include euphoria, tremors, uncoordinated action and convulsions. Indirect hazards of work at high pressure are that the effect of toxic airborne contaminants may be more severe in compressed air and emergency pressure breathing apparatus may be inadequate.

11.2   Chemical hazards

A vast number of substances present chemical hazards in the working environment. These include toxic agents having acute or chronic effects, tissue-damaging and irritant substances, asphyxiants, narcotizing and stupefying agents, carcinogens, teratogens and allergens occurring in solid, liquid, gaseous and particulate forms. The effects of these materials may be damaging to the whole body (systemic) or confined to specific parts, such as the skin, respiratory system or eyes. Some produce a range of adverse responses. In the current context, only a selection of hazardous materials can be considered. A comprehensive review is given in Sax (1979).

Toxicity of ingested materials is usefully expressed by LD_{50}, or the median lethal dose which is fatal to 50% of a large test population of experimental animals. It is specific to the type of guinea-pig used in tests and is usually normalized to units of weight of substance per weight of animal, to allow for differences amongst individuals in the test population.

The Threshold Limit Value (TLV) is a standard method of expressing toxic concentrations of chemical substances. The table of these values, published annually by the American Conference of Government Industrial Hygienists (ACGIH), defines airborne concentrations to which, it is believed, most workers may be repeatedly exposed without adverse effect. The concept includes Time Weighted Averages (TWAs), applicable to repeated exposure during a normal working week, tentative Short-Term Exposure Limits (STELs) to which workers may be exposed for periods up to 15 minutes, with no more than four such excursions per day and at least 60 minutes between them, and Ceiling Values (CV), which should never be exceeded for any period.

TLVs are derived from experience and experimental work and are supported by published material of the ACGIH, stating the sources used to define each value and the underlying objective, whether it is protection of health or comfort and amenity. They are not designed to protect individuals with above-average susceptibility, nor to form the basis for derived standards to be used in situations other than the working environment. A selection of some of the more commonly encountered hazardous chemicals is conveniently considered in groups — see Tables 11.1–11.6. The tables are not mutually exclusive and some substances are cross-referenced. The group boundaries should not, therefore, be interpreted too rigidly.

Tables 11.1–11.6   Commonly encountered hazardous chemicals.

Table 11.1   Toxic substances.

Substance	Typical sources of exposure	Effects
Metals Lead	Smelting, battery manufacture, metal recovery, crystal glass production, pigment manufacture, ceramic and paint industries. Organic compounds used in petroleum refining.	Fatigue, insomnia, headache, loss of appetite, constipation. With increased exposure, blue colouration of gum margins, abdominal cramps, severe constipation, weakening of muscles due to disturbance of the peripheral nervous system. Severe exposure can lead to encephalopathy — intense headaches, convulsions, delirium, coma, death.

continued

Table 11.1 *continued*

Substance	Typical sources of exposure	Effects
Cadmium	Metal refining, pigments, rubber and plastics additives, fungicides, photographic materials, electroplating, alloy production, battery manufacture.	Nausea, vomiting, diarrhoea, muscular cramp, salivation, kidney failure following oral ingestion. Lung irritation, chest pain, loss of sense of smell after inhalation. Implicated in bone deformations and as a carcinogen (prostate gland).
Mercury	Scientific instruments, contact breakers, chlorine production, surgical dressings, specialized paints, fungicides. The liquid metal has a high vapour pressure.	Nervous system — tremor, psychological withdrawal, irritability. Gingivitis accompanied by bluish stains on the gums. Nephrosis from acute poisoning by soluble compounds.
Zinc	Metal production, galvanizing, welding fumes.	'Metal fume fever' (not specific to zinc) from inhalation of fumes, symptoms similar to influenza.
Inorganic chemicals		
Arsenic	Pesticides, weedkillers, optical glass manufacture, anti-fouling paints, wood and fur preservatives. Sheep dip.	Irritant to mucous membranes and eyes. Highly toxic on ingestion — nervous symptoms and degeneration of the liver. Carcinogenic.
Carbon disulphide	Insecticide. Also used in varnishes, adhesives, plastics, textile treatments. Solvent of oils, fats and waxes.	Toxic to central nervous system and may lead to respiratory failure. Permanent disability may result from severe exposure.
Organic chemicals		
Benzene	Highly volatile solvent encountered in paints, resins, adhesive. Raw material for production of styrene, phenols, explosives, detergents, pharmaceuticals, dyestuffs. Constituent of motor fuel.	Chromosome aberrations possible above 25 p.p.m. Repeated exposure above 50 p.p.m. causes reduction in red blood cells, chronic exposure may lead to leukaemia. Narcotizing agent.
Xylene	Solvent in paints. Printing on plastics. Rubber industry.	Moderately toxic to blood, liver and kidneys. Narcotizing agent.
Organophosporous compounds	Malathion and related pesticides. Tricresyl phosphates, used in anti-friction oil additives and hydraulic fluids, also as additives to resins and plastics.	Lowering of blood cholinesterase, vital to the functioning of nerve cells. Pains and defective circulation in the extremities. Paralysis of limb muscles.

continued

Table 11.1   *continued*

Substance	Typical sources of exposure	Effects
Phosgene	Manufacture of dyestuffs, poly-carbonates and acid chlorides. Heating of chlorinated hydro-carbons, e.g. welding components degreased in these solvents, smoking in air contaminated by drycleaning fluids.	Serious respiratory system damage with little warning through symptoms of irritation. 50 p.p.m. in air is rapidly fatal.
2,4,5–T (2,4,5–trichlorophenoxy acetic acid)	Used as herbicide.	Highly toxic and readily ab-sorbed by inhalation/ingestion. Weakness, diarrhoea, loss of appetite, cardiac arrest and death. Reputed teratogen and carcinogen.
Gases		
Carbon monoxide	Formed during the incomplete combustion of fuels. Welding. Used in some metallurgical processes.	High affinity with haemoglobin, preventing carriage of oxygen to bodily tissues. Headache, vertigo, confusion, impairment of vision/hearing, collapse, death result from increasing concen-trations and exposure times.
Nitrous oxide	Short-duration anaesthetic. Aerosol propellant.	An experimental teratogen, sug-gested as a possible cause of abortions in operating theatre personnel.
Hydrogen cyanide	Fumigation, electroplating, synthesis of acrylonitrile.	Extremely poisonous, limiting oxygen availability to body tissues by interference with enzymes. Exposure to 100–200 p.p.m. for 30 min. may prove lethal.
Nickel carbonyl	Manufacture of pure nickel.	Irritation of respiratory tract, headache, chest pains, weakness, cyanosis. Possible carcinogen.
Hydrogen sulphide	Production of inorganic sulphides By-product of many chemical industries and may be found in enclosed spaces such as mines and sewers.	Characteristic 'bad egg' odour quickly dulls the sense of smell and enhances danger of excess exposure. Produces nausea, vertigo, irritation of respiratory system and eyes and possible nervous system disorders. High concentrations can produce death in 30 min. and very high concentrations can be immediately fatal due to paraly-sis affecting the respiratory centre.

Table 11.2   Corrosive and irritant substances

Substance	Typical sources of exposure	Effects
Acids		
Sulphuric acid	Fertilizer, drugs, dye, detergents, paper, plastics, paint manufacture. 'Pickling' iron and steel to remove rust. Battery electrolyte.	Concentrated acids present respiratory risk through fuming and serious contact hazards to skin and eyes.
Nitric acid	Fertilizer, dyestuffs, pharmaceuticals, explosives manufacture.	
Hydrochloric acid	Metal 'pickling', ammonium chloride production for manufacture of dry batteries. Soap and edible oil refining. Plastics industry.	
Hydrofluoric acid	Glass-etching, production of aerosol propellants and freons, synthesis of polytetrafluoroethylene surface coatings. Cleaning of stonework.	May penetrate skin without immediate obvious effect, but tissue destruction and possible gangrene may result. Highly irritant to mucous membranes.
Alkalis		
Sodium hydroxide (caustic soda)	Cleaning material for grease removal. Used in paper, plastics, dyestuffs, petroleum and textile industries.	Concentrated solutions strongly caustic to skin, flesh and eyes. Inhalation of dust or mists irritant and injurious to the entire respiratory tract.
Potassium hydroxide	Manufacture of liquid soap, paint strippers. Electroplating and photolithography.	
Potassium carbonate	Glass industry, engraving, tanning, pharmaceuticals.	
Gases		
Chlorine	Powerful oxidizing agent used in water disinfection. Raw material for bleach production. Manufacture of matches and chlorates for weedkiller.	Highly irritant, choking gas, forming acids with body moisture. Chronic exposure to low levels can induce permanent reduction in lung function.
Ammonia	Formation of nitrogen oxides for nitric acid manufacture. Fertilizer production. Refrigerant.	Irritant to eyes, nose, throat and skin, when liquified or in contact with moist skin.
Sulphur dioxide	Sulphuric acid production. Preservative and sterilant.	Irritant to eyes, nose and throat to such a degree that concentrations dangerous to healthy persons are easily detected.

continued

Table 11.2 *continued*

Substance	Typical sources of exposure	Effects
Nitrogen dioxide	Nitric acid production. Arc welding.	Irritation of upper respiratory tract is sometimes not severe enough to warn of serious lung damage taking place. Chronic bronchitis from long-term exposure.
Formaldehyde	Resins used in chipboard manufacture. Foam insulants. Production of Bakelite-type plastics. Disinfection and preservation.	Respiratory irritant. In solution (formalin), skin irritant and allergen. Suspected carcinogen.
Other chemicals		
Chromium and compounds	Electroplating, alloy production, pigments, wood preservation. Salts present in cement.	Ulceration of skin or nasal septum by contact or inhalation of dusts or mists. A common skin sensitizer.
Organic peroxides (particularly methyl ethyl ketone peroxide)	Hardners for polyester resins and filler pastes.	Eyes are particularly vulnerable. In bulk, these chemicals are fire and explosion hazards.

Table 11.3 Asphyxiants.

Name	Typical sources of exposure	Effects
Carbon dioxide	Combustion of fuels, welding, mines, lime kiln operations.	Displacement of air, reduces available oxygen for respiration, suffocation is possible in extreme cases.
Nitrogen	Leaks from bulk storage in connection with fertilizer production or use of nitrogen as a filler in tanks containing combustible liquids.	
Argon	Bottled gas used in welding.	

Table 11.4 Narcotizing agents.

Name	Typical sources of exposure	Effects
General		Symptoms are generally similar to those of alcohol (ethyl alcohol) intoxication, i.e. deterioration of muscle control, contraction of the peripheral field of vision, slowing of reflexes, loss of inhibitions, loss

continued

Table 11.4 *continued*

Substances	Typical sources of exposure	Effects
		of balance control, confusion, headache and slurring of speech. Coma may result from very high levels of intoxication. These effects will be present in varying degrees with the different chemicals involved. Additional effects are mentioned in this column.
Hydrocarbons		
Paraffin (kerosene)	Fuel	
White spirit	Paint thinner, cleaning solvent.	
Petrol (gasolene)	Fuel	
Benzene	(See Table 11.1)	
Toluene	Solvent capacity and occurrence similar to benzene.	
Xylene	Paints, lacquers, varnishes. Additive in aviation fuels.	
Styrene	Production of polymers (polystyrene) resins and polyesters.	Irritant to skin, mucous membranes.
Alcohols		
Ethyl alcohol (ethanol)	Evaporation from beverages stored in porous wooden casks. Synthetic rubber, plastics production.	
Methyl alcohol (methanol)	Cleaning agent. Fuel. Chemical. Feedstock.	Long elimination time from body and degrades to secondary toxic substances (formic acid, formaldehyde). Optic nerves severely affected after ingestion and blindness may result from their atrophy.
Aldehydes		
Formaldehyde	(See Table 11.2)	Some protection is afforded by irritant action on mucous membranes and eyes, compelling early removal from exposure.
Acetaldehyde	Acetic acid manufacture.	
Metaldehyde	Fuel, food additive.	
Benzaldehyde	Synthetic flavouring.	

continued

Table 11.4 *continued*

Substance	Typical sources of exposure	Effects
Ketones		
Dimethyl ketone (acetone)	Solvent in resins, lacquers, oils, fats. Used in paint, plastics, rubber, photographic industries.	Irritant action on eyes and respiratory system provides some safeguard against inhalation in narcotic concentrations. Also a potential cause of dermatitis. Ketones are rapidly excreted through the lungs and kidneys.
Diacetone alcohol	Solvent. Additive in anti-freeze, hydraulic fluids.	
Methyl ethyl ketone	Solvent for cellulose compounds. Dewaxing agents.	
Methyl-*n*-butyl ketone	Solvent in rubber, plastics, adhesives, varnishes.	
Cyclohexanone	Solvent in rubber and plastics industries.	
Ethers		
Methyl ether	Refrigerant, aerosol propellant, rocket fuel.	
Ethyl ether	Solvent for cellulose compounds, fats, gums, waxes. An early anaesthetic.	
Iso-propyl ether	Solvent in paint strippers and rubber adhesives. Additive in aviation fuels.	
Chlorinated hydrocarbons		
Trichloroethylene	Degreasing and cleaning fluids.	Carbon tetrachloride has largely been replaced by others in this group, on account of its toxicity.
Tetrachlorethylene		
Carbon tetrachloride		
Alpha-trichloroethane	Solvent in typewriter correction fluid.	
Numerous pesticides	Pest control.	Other toxic effects.

Table 11.5 Carcinogens.

Name	Typical sources of exposure	Effects
Natural materials		
Wood dusts	Furniture industries, wood turning. Beech and African hardwood specifically implicated.	Cancer of the nasal passages.

continued

Table 11.5   *continued*

Substance	Typical sources of exposure	Effects
Asbestos	Friction linings, insulants, gasket and linoleum manufacture, building products.	Mesothelioma of pleural/peritoneal cavities is characteristic. Lung cancer. Asbestosis (see Chap. 6).
Manufactured materials		
Tar, pitch	Fuel briquetting, water proofing, construction industries.	Epitheliomata on hands, arms, neck, head or scrotum.
Cutting oils	Lubricants/coolants used during metal machining.	Cancer of hands, forearms, scrotum, the latter being particularly at risk when contaminated clothing is worn for extended periods.
Lead chromate	Chrome yellow pigment, liable to be inhaled during spraying operations.	Lung cancer.
Vinyl chloride	Gaseous monomer for the polymerization of PVC.	Angiosarcoma of the liver. Also highly inflammable and a skin irritant.
Cadmium	(See Table 11.1).	Increased incidence of prostatic cancer after long-term occupational exposure. Acute respiratory and other effects described in Table 11.1.
Methylene-bis-ortho-chloroaniline	Curing agent in the production of rigid polyurethane foams and the moulding of urethane rubber articles.	Experimental carcinogen (liver and lung tumours) in rats. Skin irritant.
Alpha-naphthylamine	Rubber manufacture, used under strictly controlled conditions to improve durability.	Bladder cancer. A less potent carcinogen than beta-naphthlyamine, prohibited in the U.K. since 1967 but which may still occur as an impurity in alpha-naphthylamine.

Table 11.6   Allergens/sensitizers.

Name	Typical sources of exposure	Effects
White spirit	Manufacture, use as cleaning material, paint thinner.	Dermatitis, notably of the hands, following the removal of natural oils from the skin.

continued

Table 11.6 *continued*

Substance	Typical sources of exposure	Effects
Chlorinated hydrocarbons (trichloroethylene, carbon tetrachloride, etc.)	Cleaning and degreasing fluids.	As above. Also narcotizing agents.
Mineral oils	Fuels, lubricants. Oil mists from compressors and air tools.	Oil acne, dermatitis.
Toluene diisocyanate	Manufacture of polyurethane foams, paints, printing on plastic materials, specialized fabric treatments.	An irritant which may precipitate asthma. Long exposure may sensitize skin and cause dermatitis.
Washing powders	Manufacture and use.	Dermatitis.
Wood dusts	Furniture industries.	Skin sensitization, dermatitis. Also respiratory irritants, causing rhinitis, asthma. Some varieties carcinogenic.
Nickel	Handling cupro-nickel coinage.	Nickel dermatitis.
Coal tar products		
Pitch	Battery manufacture.	Dermatitis
Phenols	Disinfectants.	
Cresols	Adhesives, disinfectants.	
Cotton	Textile, rope production.	Byssinosis, a progressive, chronic bronchitis contracted through inhalation of particulate matter from these products. It is not entirely agreed whether this is a true allergic reaction or the result of repeated irritation.
Flax		
Hemp		

Exposure to chemical hazards is a much more frequent occurrence in industrial occupations than in office or shop work, but commercial premises are not exempt from these risks. The open-plan office presents many advantages to the business organization seeking economy in space and partitioning and flexibility in building use. However this type of construction, made possible by structural engineering advances, lends itself readily to environmental conditioning by sophisticated heating, ventilation and air-conditioning systems in buildings which become virtually sealed capsules, where a variety of substances whose effects are only partly known, for example solvents from type-correcting fluids, fire-retardants, cleaning materials, adhesives, air-fresheners, etc. are introduced and circulated.

11.3 Protection against chemicals and particulates

Protection against chemical hazards is a specialized field of activity in its own right. The promotion of safety rests on the basic policies of (*i*) substitution of less dangerous materials; (*ii*) enclosure of processes; (*iii*) controlled exposure; and (*iv*) personal protection.

11.3.1   Substitution

Substitution is an attractive proposition on health protection grounds and for economic reasons, where it can obviate the need for expensive monitoring and control procedures.It is this philosophy which has led to the preference of other less toxic solvents to benzene, where practicable, and it seems likely that the insulation industry will turn increasingly to the use of mineral fibres other than asbestos, having regard to the elaborate safety precautions which are necessary during its installation, removal and disposal. Already, the importation of blue asbestos (crocidolite) into the U.K. has been prohibited, forcing the choice of alternative materials. Substitution is, however, unlikely ever to be applicable to more than a very small minority of chemicals used in industry.

11.3.2   Enclosure

Enclosure of industrial processes can present severe practical difficulties in maintaining access to the work in progress and achieving reasonable speed of production but has, nevertheless, been highly developed in some places. The increasing use of robot machinery in Japan and elsewhere opens up possibilities for progressive separation of men and hazardous processes. Where the most stringent isolation of processes is not necessary, it is still sound practice to group moderately hazardous exposure sources together, so that their effects are largely confined to one part of the premises and can be dealt with by an integrated, rather than fragmented, control system. Segregation of personnel can be considered as another aspect of enclosure, only in this case it is the workers who are contained in a control room or similar structure, shielded from physical exposure to the hazardous material and supplied with air under positive pressure from a clean source, yet still able to supervise automated processes.

11.3.3   Control of exposure

Control of exposure starts with a good standard of basic cleanliness, followed by careful design of buildings and plant. Examples illustrating unnecessary exposure, almost totally avoidable by proper attention to these requirements, are still to be seen in poorly managed workplaces — bad planning of work layout and slack cleaning routines permitting toxic matter to be trodden from place to place, contaminated working clothes worn in canteens, spent process materials left to fume in the open air, affecting passers by.

Mechanical dust suppression is an important safety system in many industries and should be designed to prevent, as far as possible, the escape of particulate from the immediate process area into the general work room environment. Receptor hoods are designed to receive dust-laden air, driven into the hood by some feature of the process. The captor hood is intended to have a more positive effect, by drawing in contaminated air which would otherwise tend to disperse, by the suction of a powerful fan which overcomes the outward motion of the airborne particles. It may be assisted by appropriately placed air jets. Both systems are connected to ducts, the contents of which are propelled to a point of external discharge, which must be selected to prevent a secondary pollution problem. Dust cleaning may well be necessary before the stream is emitted to the atmosphere. Very careful design and maintenance are necessary to ensure the effective performance of these systems. Poor design can easily worsen problems by distributing the contaminant and maintenance should only be undertaken by personnel fully familiar with the objective and operating principles of the installation.

Portable power tools can be a source of considerable dust emission and somewhat similar principles can be applied to its control. Extractor heads can be fitted to many tools and rely on accurate design, construction and fitting to create an air current which, whilst of low volume, has a high suction velocity near the working tip of the tool. A remote turbo-exhauster can serve several of these units through flexible hose connections.

Where dust arises from multiple sources distributed over a wide area, treatment of the general workroom atmosphere may be called for. Available techniques include filtration, water scrubbing and electrostatic precipitation. Selection of the appropriate technique should be based on knowledge of the dust burden and its relative toxicity. Dilution ventilation is a less effective method of dust abatement, by diluting its concentration with incoming fresh air, rather than removing the dust. The general principles of dust control are applicable to numerous situations in which fumes and vapours are involved.

Control of exposure to liquid and solid substances involves some degree of automated handling to reduce the possibilities of contact between people and materials. In the context of protection against the physical hazard of ionizing radiation, such systems have been highly developed to deal with the remote handling of spent power station fuel elements containing high-activity radionuclides.

Time is an important factor in the control of exposure and Threshold Limit Values (see p. 169) are very much concerned with time and concentration taken together in assessing the acceptability of work in contaminated surroundings.

11.3.4 Personal protection

Personal protection is not as attractive an option as those of substitution and enclosure. Training is required in the use and limitations of protective equipment, there are sometimes problems in ensuring that it is used, personal fitting is required and a regular maintenance system is essential. All these points introduce risk of failure through human error.

Respirators provide defence against airborne contaminants, provided that they are correctly fitted and matched to the requirements for protection. Gases and particulates require different techniques of removal and the particle size and burden of dusts may be critical. The increased resistance to airflow makes work carried out whilst wearing the respirator more tiring, and there is thus some temptation to discard it, unless warning of necessity is given by the visibility of a hazard, an air monitoring instrument or detection through the sense of smell. Pressurized breathing apparatus can be bulky and cumbersome in use, but provides an increased margin of safety over filter-based methods, particularly when working with highly toxic substances or atmospheres which may be oxygen-deficient, and gains some advantage in reduced airflow resistance. Negative-pressure systems, which rely on the intermittent provision of air in response to the partial vacuum created by the act of inspiration, are susceptible to inleakage and should be discarded in favour of positive-pressure apparatus which removes this danger by providing a constant pressurized supply. Breathing apparatus which relies on bottled air supplies must be carefully monitored to ensure sufficient reserves are maintained and increased safety, at the expense of mobility, is obtained by using an external source of clean air delivered by an air hose.

Eye protection needs to be specific to the type of hazard involved as different performance is required in the case of chemicals, high velocity impacts and molten metals.

Overalls have an important safety function, being frequently the first line of defence of the skin against hazardous materials, as well as preventing the soiling of other clothing. Regular cleaning is essential to prevent the gradual migration of harmful substances through layers of clothing. The risk of skin cancer, particularly of the scrotum, caused by prolonged contact with clothing saturated with mineral oils used in metal machining operations, is sufficiently well known to give heavy emphasis to this point.

Gloves provide a barrier between the skin and irritant or corrosive substances, as well as heat, flames and sparks. When selected for protection against chemicals, choice of type and composition must have regard to the relative caustic or solvent properties of the process material and the degree of risk should the gloves be punctured or become impervious. When handling materials such as hydrofluoric acid, serious injuries have resulted from the penetration of a very small quantity of the acid. Dermatitis may be aggravated rather than prevented by the entry of a small amount of allergenic material into gloves, which is then kept in continous contact with the skin. Certain types of rubber contain substances which are themselves irritant and a cause of hand-eczema. Barrier creams may provide the only effective protection where gloves would seriously impede manual dexterity or create the risk of entrapment in moving machinery.

11.4   Microbiological hazards

Microbiological infections are associated with many occupations, so specifically in some cases that they are colloquially described by reference to that trade or profession, for instance, 'Farmers Lung' (see below and Chap. 6).

Anthrax, once readily contracted by people in contact with live infected animals or their meat and by-products, has been greatly reduced in incidence through the routine disinfection of by-products and the rigorous disinfection procedures (including on the spot slaughter and carcase incineration) applied after diagnosis in animals. Most cases which do occur are contracted via the skin, during the handling of hides, leading to the formation of a pustule 1–8 days later. In this form (hide-carrier's disease), the condition responds to antibiotic or serum treatment. Pulmonary anthrax (wool-sorter's disease) occurs as a result of inhalation of the bacilli and, after an incubation period of 2–6 days, progresses rapidly with fever and acute respiratory effects leading to very high mortality rates. Infection by the gastrointestinal route is also possible. Spores of the causal organisms, *Bacillus anthracis*, are very long-lived and highly resistant to extremes of temperature and dehydration and may survive hostile conditions for many years.

Tuberculosis has now been brought largely under control in developed countries, in both man and animals, by sustained public health and veterinary campaigns. As an occupational disease, it is still liable to be acquired in poorer parts of the world by a combination of poor general health and unhygienic conditions. The unskilled, undernourished and badly housed are at greatest risk, particularly when employed in polluted conditions which affect the health of the lungs, providing a site for the settlement of airborne bacilli, more readily available in overcrowded and poorly ventilated premises. Skin infection may be contracted in farming, veterinary and butchery occupations.

Brucellosis, the cause of contagious abortion in cattle, with similar organisms affecting other food, domestic and wild animals, has been the subject of a well advanced eradication scheme in Britain (Chap. 3), but remains endemic in some countries where it is the cause of serious economic loss. The primary routes of human infection are contact, inhalation and ingestion by those exposed to infected animals or animal by-products and the disease is often characterized by fever, with weakness in the joints and muscles, together with pain, although symptoms can be highly variable. Whilst of low mortality, the disease in humans is distressing because symptoms may recur after apparent recovery over a long period. For this reason it is popularly described as undulant fever.

Weil's disease (leptospirosis) principally affects rodents, but there are possibilities of occupational exposure in work associated with animal contact or exposure to sewage. The causal organism is a slender spirochaete, which gains access to the body via skin abrasions or mucous membranes and, after an incubation period of some 7–10 days, produces symptoms which vary considerably in severity. Fever, muscle pains, headache, loss of appetite, nausea, profuse sweating and disruption of bowel function may be experienced. The liver is frequently affected, with consequent jaundice, and there may be some involvement of the respiratory and central nervous systems. In severe cases, kidney failure may lead to death. Rodent control in general, and especially in sewers, has greatly assisted in the control of this disease and its incidence had been reduced to 103 confirmed cases in the two-year period 1979–80 (Leptospira Reference Library).

The *animal population*, as a reservoir of numerous conditions transmissible to man, is discussed in Chap. 3 and farmers, abattoir workers and others handling live animals or meat and animal by-products obviously face the most immediate risks from exposure to such hazards. Raw meat must always be regarded as a potential carrier of pathogens which may not have produced ante-mortem symptoms or visible lesions in the carcase and offal. Cuts and abrasions to the hands are acknowledged routes of infecting food (see Chap. 8), and may also provide a means for the entry of pathogens into the body.

The *fungal diseases*, or *mycoses*, can be occupationally acquired. 'Athlete's foot', verrucae and other diseases affecting the skin, and thus spread by contact, are a risk to people whose work exposes them to wet conditions shared communally, such as factory or pithead showers and changing rooms. Other mycoses affect deeper structures of the body and may be spread in the bloodstream after inoculation or inhalation. Aspergillosis (Farmer's lung), which may result from the inhalation of spores contained in mouldy hay or other vegetable material, referred to in Chap. 6, is a prescribed disease under industrial injuries legislation.

Medical and nursing personnel are exposed to a whole range of pathogens carried by the patients whom they attend. Viral hepatitis has become a significant disease amongst medical staff in recent years and is particularly associated with renal dialysis units, where the viruses may easily be acquired orally, or by inoculation from the blood of an infected patient.

11.5   Mental and social factors

It is increasingly recognized that mental health at work is not merely concerned with the diagnosis and treatment of clinically recognized conditions, but also with the creation of a positively healthy environment. Subclinical unhealthiness is not always immediately apparent in a person's mental state, any more than it is in his physical condition. The decline from good health is often an insidious process and, after a while, accepted (if it is recognized at all) as the normal state of life. An unknown proportion of the adult population probably suffers from minor psychological symptoms which are unlikely ever to prompt them to seek professional assistance. To the observer, these people are likely to present no more than evidence of common personality factors — aggressiveness, withdrawal, suspicion of others, accident-proneness — developed to an unusual degree. In more noticeable cases suspicions may be aroused as a result of more pronounced behavioural disorders, such as alcoholism.

The practice of good management is rarely recognized as a function to promote the mental well-being of people at work, yet often has identical objectives. Both are concerned with the relationships between the individual and his or her employing organization, actual tasks, and fellow workers. Both should recognize that the successful functioning of the organization depends on the correct handling of the human resource. Neglect of this principle, apart from the cost in human terms, is increasingly accepted as a recipe for dissatisfaction, demotivation, absenteeism, low productivity and labour disputes.

Rivalry between peers, in moderation, is a normal manifestation of working life, as it is in competitive sports. If it is allowed to develop to the point of actions damaging to the status, reputation or promotion prospects of others, an unhealthy situation has been created, which is enhanced if the conflict is in a senior *versus* junior context. It is not infrequently felt by junior staff that they are more capable than their superiors and such sentiments, if kept within reasonable limits, may be identified as ambition leading eventually to the promotion which is desired. If they are expressed in over-vigorous terms, retaliation is usually provoked by the blocking of the junior's promotion or his or her transfer to some less desirable task or work location. Some managers, with a strong dislike of their own inadequacies, do not need provocation to behave in this way. They constantly try to shift the burden of their own failings onto their subordinates by hostile criticism, undermining their confidence in their capabilities and blaming them for all the failures of the organization. They stand in contrast to the confident and secure manager who encourages the development of his or her juniors and is keen to promote their mental health by exposing talent which, perhaps, they themselves did not know they possessed.

11.5.1   Stress and strain

Stress and strain — terms borrowed from engineering vocabulary denoting the load placed on a body and its effect — have been accused of contributing to many types of ill-health, particularly mental ill-health, and have been identified in many types of occupation. They are particularly associated with work which is always carried out against time schedules, accompanied by frequent interruptions or when handling several complicated tasks at the same time — consider the air traffic controller's heavy responsibilities at a busy international airport in bad weather. Patterns of work are also relevant. The human system appears to function best in stable and regular programmes of activity and to require a fairly lengthy period of adjustment after changes in these routines. 'Jet-lag' is experienced when people travel rapidly across the world's time zones and, for a while, their personal time 'clock' is out of phase with the local times of waking, sleeping and eating. Much the same effects are complained of by workers changing their shifts of duties so frequently that the body is unable to become attuned to the changes. This familiar cause of dissatisfaction can be alleviated by arranging much longer intervals between changes of regular shifts.

Any situation in life seen as a threat to the ambitions, safety or well-being of the individual constitutes stress, whether consciously recognized as such, or not. Physical reactions are measurable in the nervous and endocrine systems of the body and are designed to increase the capability of defence against or flight from the hostile situation. Longlasting or repeated stress situations can lead to permanent changes in the functions of parts of the body and are suggested as a possible cause of eventual impairment of those functions. They take their rise from aggressive supervision, threats to the achievement of goals, deterioration in the physical environment, quarrels with colleagues and a multitude of other incidents and patterns of behaviour. They produce varying reactions in different individuals and at different times in the same individual.

Suitability for the job is a matter of prime importance. The person promoted beyond his or her capabilities is frequently assailed by anxieties about his or her incapacity, manifested typically by depression and the development of unfounded concern with physical health. Underwork is also mentally damaging and may be interpreted as lack of trust by superiors, leading ultimately to deteriorating self-confidence and the gradual impoverishment of personality.

11.5.2   General fatigue

General fatigue is a condition characterized by loss of energy, depression and lowering of initiative accompanied by psychosomatic disturbances such as insomnia, headaches, loss of appetite, cardiac and digestive disorders. As the causative factors may be physical and mental, it may be considered to be a further demonstration of the concept of health as a combination of favourable physical, mental and social conditions. Physical causes contributing to general fatigue include noise, light, heat, air quality and comfort of surroundings. The mental causes are likely to be worry, conflict, monotony, pressure of responsibilities and lack of regular breaks. The common experience of fatigue has been demonstrated in physiological studies showing that repeated stimulation of certain centres of the brain gradually reduces the capacity for performance and periods of rest are necessary for the restoration of peak response, by allowing the activating systems of the brain to regain dominance over their inhibitory rivals. The situation is, in fact, analogous to physical fatigue, where rest of the body is necessary for the replenishment of muscle tissue.

Part IV Protection and Prevention

12
Safeguarding the environment

12.1 Introduction

The environment in which we live is determined partly by geography and climate, but also by human activity. The problems which may result from overcrowding, bad housing, inadequate food, space and light, dirty water supplies, inappropriate sewage disposal, and pollution by domestic and industrial detritus, were discussed in Chap. 2, and illustrated by reference to the effects of the industrial revolution. This aspect of the environment is susceptible to legislative control and legal enforcement and, indeed, vast improvements have been brought about by such means during the last two centuries. A continuous programme of observation, surveillance and enforcement, associated with research and the implementation of new measures to deal more effectively with old hazards or combat new ones is necessary (Fig. 12.1). British legislation has a long history of imposing the duty of

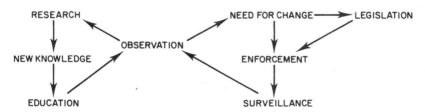

Fig. 12.1 Safeguarding the macroenvironment.

surveillance on workers in the environmental health field, traditionally employed by local authorities. The Public Health Act 1848 created a General Board of Health with local subordinate boards, each of which was required to appoint an Inspector of Nuisances who, working under the 'general direction of the Medical Officer of Health' was required 'by inspection of his district . . . to keep himself informed of the sanitary circumstances of the district . . .'. The modern equivalent of early public health law makes extensive similar provision (Table 12.1).

Since 1974, the Medical Officer of Health, formerly employed by the Local Authority and responsible for all aspects of the public health scene, has been

Table 12.1 Examples of the duty of environmental surveillance placed on authorities in the United Kingdom.

Duty of local authority to inspect its area to detect noise nuisances (Section 57(a), Contro of Pollution Act, 1974).

Power of the Health and Safety Commission to direct a report to be made on 'any accident, occurrence, situation or other matter whatsoever' (Section 14(2)(a), Health and Safety at Work Act, 1974).

Duty of local authority to 'cause an inspection of their district to be made from time to time with a view to ascertaining whether any house therein is unfit for human habitation' (Section 3, Housing Act, 1957).

Power of local authority to undertake air pollution investigation and research (Section 79, Control of Pollution Act, 1974).

---

replaced by the 'Medical Officer for Environmental Health'. This officer is employed by the Health Authority in the locality, and seconded for part of his time to give medical support and advice to the District Council and its environmental health officers who now work under the direction of a Chief Environmental Health Officer who is accountable to the Council (see Table 12.2). Clinics, ambulance services and other personal health services which had developed in the local authority context under the guidance of medical officers of health passed to the control of the new Health Authorities in 1974, leaving the more technical environmental health services with the local authority.

Monitoring the environment is an important part of a strategy to safeguard it by comparing the situation which does exist with that which should exist. The system recognizes the importance of both inspections and actual measurement of environmental quality factors using scientific methods (see Fig. 12.2 and 12.5). Some of the techniques adopted were described in part III of this book. Results can be compared with criteria recognized as being compatible with public health and safety, or with reference levels found in other areas. Trends in pollution levels may be monitored (see Figs 12.3, 12.4); levels which might not be considered

Table 12.2 Local agencies concerned with aspects of the environment in the United Kingdom.

	Environmental Health Officer	Medical Officer for Environmental Health	Scientific Adviser	Regional Water Authority	Public Health Laboratory
Housing	+	−	0	0	0
Food	+	+	+	0	+
Noise	+	+	−	0	0
Water	+	+	+	+	+
Air	+	+	+	0	0
Safety	+	−	−	0	0
Communicable disease	+	+	0	−	+

+ Major involvement
− Minor involvement
0 No involvement

hazardous on contemporary information may be questioned as the results of further research emerge. Monitoring can assist in the evaluation of proposals to develop land or install new plant in existing premises by establishing ambient pollution levels so as to determine the impact of a new pollutant source and whether it can be accommodated without unacceptable environmental deterioration. The need for improved emission controls may be demonstrated by monitoring, also the effectiveness of controls when they have been introduced. The data obtained may lead either to action following the justification of complaints or the withdrawal of complaints shown to be unfounded.

12.2   Air pollution monitoring

Systematic measurement of air pollution in the United Kingdom dates back to 1914. By 1981, over 1000 installations were being used for daily smoke and sulphur dioxide observations, using standardized apparatus in a national survey coordinated by the Department of Industry's Warren Spring Laboratory (Fig. 12.2). Results obtained using such apparatus are shown in Figs 12.3 and 12.4. The specifications for the methods are laid down in parts two and three of British Standard 1747: 1969. Air pollution control is a multidisciplinary activity. Monitoring the general environment is, together with the enforcement of the Clean Air and Control of Pollution Acts as they apply to domestic and the less complex industrial premises, a

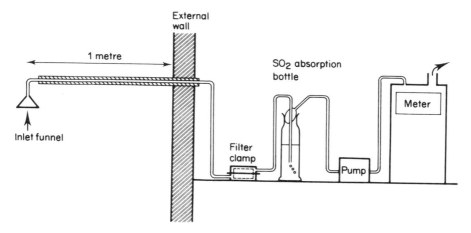

Fig. 12.2   Schematic representation of volumetric apparatus for the determination of smoke and sulphur dioxide in air.

function of District Councils. The more sophisticated and large-scale industrial installations, such as chemical and metallurgical process works and power stations, are, with few exceptions, scheduled under the Health and Safety (Emissions into the Atmosphere) Regulations 1983, made under the Health and Safety at Work Act 1974. Under this system, prior approval, periodical inspection and registration are the responsibility of Her Majesty's Industrial Air Pollution Inspectorate of the Health and Safety Executive. Approval to commission and operate these works is conditional on employment of the 'best practicable means' to limit

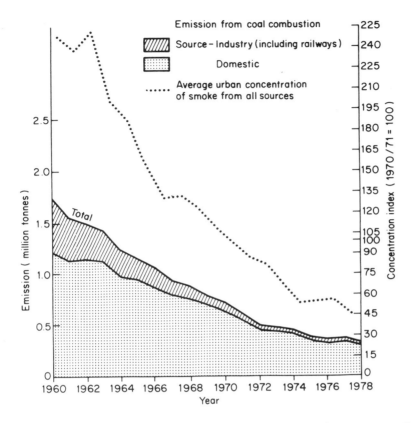

Fig. 12.3 Smoke: trends in emissions and average urban concentrations in the United Kingdom. (Crown copyright. Reproduced by permission of the Director, Warren Spring Laboratory, Department of Industry.)

the discharge of noxious or offensive materials to the atmosphere. The system is flexible and, since full advantage can be taken of the latest developments in emission control when the requirements for re-registration are decided, encourages a continuing improvement in air quality. The preference for rigid criteria displayed generally in Europe and North America has the advantage of defining targets more specifically, but fresh legislation is needed each time a further stage of improvement is sought.

The enforcement agencies receive expert scientific support through the activities of the Government Chemist (serving the Health and Safety Executive) and County Scientific Advisers (undertaking analytical and other work for District Councils) (see Table 12.2). Basic and applied research undertaken by Warren Spring Laboratory, Universities and associations financed by industry, makes an important contribution to a deeper understanding of air pollution problems. When all organizations concerned work together, the prospect of successful programmes of improvement is greatly enhanced. The results of the cooperative approach can be seen in the work of such organizations as the Bristol and District Environmental

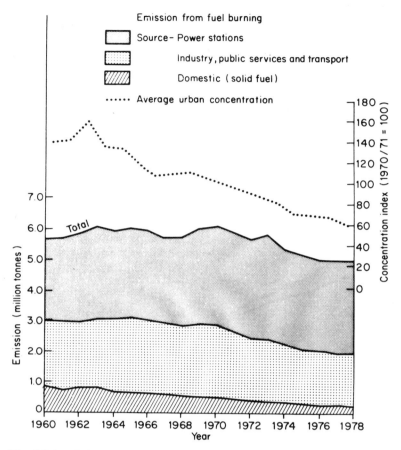

Fig. 12.4   Sulphur dioxide: trends in emissions and average urban concentrations in the United Kingdom. (Crown copyright. Reproduced by permission of the Director, Warren Spring Laboratory, Department of Industry.)

Pollution Technical Committee, the Coventry Pollution Prevention Panel and the Greater Manchester Council for Clean Air.

12.3   Housing

Political commitment to improvement of the environment is nowhere more important than in the sphere of housing policy. Housing is an inherently expensive commodity and the provision of an ample supply of accommodation, situated in areas of demand, well-equipped and properly maintained, requires the devotion of a substantial share of the community's wealth. Ideological differences as to the relative merits of various types of tenure and systems of finance have all too often been concerned merely with the details of distribution of resources, rather than ensuring that their size is adequate for the justified claims made upon them. Successive shifts in emphasis have done little to promote long-term stability.

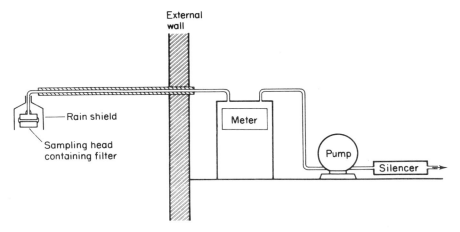

Fig. 12.5   Sampling equipment for metals in air.

Whilst progress has been made with some aspects of housing improvement (see p. 156), there is no room for complacency in the knowledge that more than 1 in 10 of the population are living in conditions which are unsatisfactory, either because of disrepair or lack of amenities in their homes. This judgement is made on the basis of current standards and it is surely reasonable that these should be increased in the future to take account of the external environment, storage space, fire safety, heating systems, privacy, sound insulation between dwellings and the accommodation of domestic appliances such as freezers and washing machines now owned by substantial numbers of the population. If and when housing criteria rise to meet the expectations created by the general increase in material prosperity an even greater proportion of homes will be found to fall short in one way or another.

There are now marginally more homes available than households to occupy them, but this national average statistic should not obscure pockets of serious regional shortage. Housing stress is still most acutely felt in London, where, although the overall population has decreased, the number of households has not, and large numbers of people occupy accommodation which is in some part shared, of necessity rather than by choice. Inadequacy of maintenance has led to the eventual loss of many houses in London and their replacement is slowed by insufficiency of funds. At the other extreme, a significant amount of under-occupation persists in large houses suitable for division into flats, but remaining unconverted because of restricted opportunities for recovering the costs via rent income. The personal tragedy of homelessness afflicts many people, frequently resulting from the dissolution of households after the breakdown of marriage. An estimated 273 000 homes are needed for single people in Scotland (Scottish Council for Single Homeless, 1981, *Think Single*) yet there is reason to believe that many single people in housing need do not apply for local authority accommodation, believing their chances of success too remote.

The housing environment changes so rapidly that it is of the greatest importance for it to be monitored at frequent intervals, so that changing needs and developing problems will be identified. It is only by the provision of such intelligence that determination to solve the problems will be engendered and maintained.

Unfortunately, the surveys needed to provide this information are costly in terms of manpower and they are a tempting target for expenditure restrictions forced on public authorities, but they are as essential to the treatment of housing problems as diagnosis is to medical care.

The provision of housing subsidies appears to correlate poorly with individual needs, substantial benefit being available to relatively affluent owner-occupiers, in the form of tax-relief on mortgage interest, and to many local authority tenants where subsidy is largely attached to the house, rather than the occupants, whilst very limited help is available to some of the poorest sections of the community renting accommodation privately. In an economy where the share of public expenditure allotted to housing was 10% in 1974, but expected to be only just over 4% by 1984, this situation calls for examination and perhaps the institution of a unified housing benefit directly related to the needs of individuals.

12.4   Food hygiene and control

Although notable improvements in food hygiene have occurred in the past, such as the virtual eradication of tuberculosis and brucellosis from milk, there is still much to be done. For instance, the number of reported food poisoning cases in England and Wales showed an unwelcome increase of about 60% between 1970 and 1981, and increases have also been observed in other European countries. Statistics are always confounded by unreported incidents and the figures may partly reflect an increased willingness to seek medical attention and improved diagnostic procedures resulting in a greater number of cases being brought to the attention of local authorities. However, the occurrence of over 13 000 reported cases in 1981 cannot be regarded as a satisfactory situation, although it is some improvement on the peak of over 14 000 recorded in 1979.

It is generally a difficult matter to prove a direct relationship between food poisoning statistics and the prevalence of bad practices or the introduction of new techniques of food handling and processing. Similarly, the detection of the source of individual cases is an exercise which meets with mixed success. The usual procedure is to take a careful medical history, since the symptomatology of the case will often give an initital indication of the most likely causative agent. This is followed by an equally careful history of recent food consumption, giving particular attention to those foods which are known to be most associated with food poisoning. Bacteriological and virological investigations of the case and suspect food stuffs may follow. Speed of diagnosis, notification and investigation is essential, as important evidence contained in food remnants and containers is quickly disposed of and memories of the content of meals soon fade. The causes of outbreaks of food poisoning present a better prospect of successful detection. Where a number of people have been infected with the same strain of organism, careful questioning and recording has a better chance of identifying common factors in the recent eating patterns of the patients and pointing to a shared source of infection which can be investigated in depth.

The two principal strategies for food protection are education and enforcement. Without a vast increase in the number of environmental health officers no more than sporadic visits can be made to each of the hundreds of thousands of food handling establishments in Britain and they may be made at times not wholly representative of actual trading conditions. Furthermore, a policy limited to enforcement does very little to promote a true understanding of the principles of hygiene. It is far too easy to accept the superficial features of premises as presenting the total picture and to ignore the important part played by good systems of food handling and an awareness by staff of the significance of their personal actions. There exist many premises in which, from experience, the proprietors have learned to provide the necessary washbasins, refrigerators and 'no-smoking' notices to ward off the unwelcome attentions of the environmental health department, but in which the unseen actions and omissions in preparation rooms away from the public gaze may be dubious in the extreme.

Basic education in bacteriology and hygiene is therefore extremely important in the campaign for safe food and it is to be hoped that these subjects will form an area of increasing interest in the training of food handlers. Education of the public is equally important, since they are responsible for the treatment of food once it has left the retailers' premises. Despite numerous warnings, there are still cases of food poisoning attributable to the cooking of insufficiently thawed frozen poultry and it is not uncommon to see high-risk products — pies, pâté and the like — incubating in the back of private cars after purchase on sunny days.

Whatever the benefits of education, there must remain an enforcement role for public authorities. In any commercial activity there will be a minority of operators who are concerned only with maximum gain, untroubled by considerations of public protection and safety unless threatened with penal sanctions. The salutary effect of a well-publicized prosecution is readily observable in this small, otherwise less-responsive group. In 1980 it became clear that illicit trading in unfit and diseased meat was increasing in certain parts of Britain, no doubt prompted by the high profit obtainable by the clandestine acquisition of such material and its disguise by trimming, superficial cleaning and incorporation in made-up products. A high degree of certainty of detection and the imposition of heavy penalties are needed to end this dangerous practice.

The large numbers of people and premises involved in food handling suggests that some system of risk assessment and priority classification is needed. There are a number of ways in which this can be done. One approach is to grade all food premises according to the type of product handled, allocating the lowest risk category to undertakings concerned only with wrapped food or raw vegetables and the highest to those dealing with foods highly conducive to bacterial growth. The potential number of consumers affected by the establishment may also be relevant. For instance, 50 to 100 cattle might be slaughtered each working day in a busy abattoir, each carcase weighing some 250 kg and representing 2000 or so individual portions of meat. The scale of such an operation has obvious significance in setting and achieving the necessary standards of hygiene. Priority may also be identified by a system involving the allocation of points having regard to the condition of premises, freedom from practices likely to lead to contamination, the effectiveness of cleaning plans and adequacy of staff training. When totalled and divided into a 'weighting' factor determined by the relative risk of the activity undertaken, a relative degree of risk is determined, which approximates to the amount of concern and activity necessary at those premises (see Roberts, 1980). Whilst these systems are inevitably subject to some degree of uncertainty and variation, they are a significant improvement on purely arbitrary approaches to the subject.

The application of microbiological standards to food is a matter which is subject to some controversy, although some authorities are now starting to enact limits on the types and number of bacteria present in certain foods intended for retail sale. There are difficulties in ensuring that samples taken to check compliance are, by the time they have been transported to the laboratory and waited for examination, still representative of the condition of the food at the time of sale and this policy needs to be developed with caution. Bacteriological sampling under the controlled conditions of the factory environment is a useful method of indicating the need for more detailed investigation of the production chain where adverse results are obtained at any point. Simple tests, such as the methylene blue test for milk and ice-cream have long been in use as general indicators of bacteriological quality. Swabbing of work surfaces and equipment can be a valuable supplement to visual inspections of premises in pinpointing the places where bacteria are harboured, identifying the areas where improved cleaning routines are needed.

The Department of Health and Social Security plays an important part in advising District Councils in the discharge of their food control functions and the Public Health Laboratory Service undertakes essential microbiological investigations to support the field work of inspection and sampling. A similar role is carried out in respect of chemical composition by County Scientific Advisers. Trading Standards, or Consumer Protection Officers are also concerned, amongst many other matters, with food, their particular emphasis being placed on the protection of quality and labelling, more than on health. The whole area of food control thus provides another example of the need for effective teamwork.

12.5   Water quality

The abundance of water in nature has, in the past, led to abuse of natural sources, but the vastly increased demands of industrial societies have shown that water is a resource demanding proper management. Analytical equipment has been developed to advanced standards of sensitivity and there are now few problems in monitoring water quality with speed and accuracy. Technical developments in treatment have needed to keep pace with the increasing use of complex chemical compounds which are liable to find their way into waste water and have also been triggered by the economics of recycling. As environmental quality standards have been made more stringent and improved effluent treatment becomes necessary, it has been increasingly attractive for industry to invest a little extra to upgrade the effluent for re-use as process water.

The rate of biological filtration, previously determined by the characteristics of the traditional materials used in the filter beds, has been improved by the use of plastic media. Because of higher initial cost, a greater loading of the media is required and two or three sequential treatments may be needed to secure quality comparable with that of conventional systems. A number of improvements to the activated sludge process employing high concentrations and transfer rates of dissolved oxygen with energy consumption not exceeding that of conventional plants have been developed in recent years.

Government policy has kept pace with the need for greater care over the conservation of water resources and major legislation (the Water Act 1973) unified the functions of control over the provision and use of supplies, effluent treatment, river improvement and inland navigation. The operation of the Act is principally in the hands of Regional Water Authorities (see Table 12.2), acting under the guidance of a National Water Council which reports to the Secretary of State for the Environment.

12.6   Occupational health

Occupational health administration in Britain has been radically altered by the Health and Safety at Work Act, 1974, which, by stages, is bringing together and updating former legislation under a new and comprehensive policy designed to promote safe working conditions and practices. The emphasis is being changed fundamentally from that of a fragmented system of regulatory enactments, in which safety was seen mainly as a matter of rectifying specific situations defined by the law as dangerous, to a much more positive concept, identifying safety and welfare as tangible benefits to be achieved through commitment and effort. Some of the important features of the legislation are the right of employees to appoint their own safety representatives, with responsibilities for identifying hazards at work, and the individual liabilities placed on managers for ensuring safe working practices.

Enforcement is the responsibility of the Health and Safety Executive (in general, as regards industrial activities) and local authorities (dealing mainly with non-industrial work, e.g. shop, office, educational work). The strategy for dealing with safety problems is in the hands of the Health and Safety Commission, an independant authority for which the Secretary of State is answerable to Parliament, although he is not involved in the detailed management of the Commission. Its work includes the preparation of codes of practice for safe work, research, advice, the promotion of education and training and preparing revisions and additions to legislation.

Legislation imposes the basic requirement on employers to provide a healthy and safe working environment, with safe systems of work and healthy premises with sufficient amenities. They are also obliged to prepare, and keep updated, a written safety policy which must be brought to the attention of all employees and demonstrate how hazards will be identified and treated. Employees have a duty to exercise due care for their own safety, and that of their fellows, and not to interfere with or misuse anything provided in the interests of health, safety and welfare.

As safety-consciousness amongst both employers and staff representatives develops, it is to be expected that the demand for education will grow and will be coupled with an increase in requirements for more factual information based on monitoring of the working environment. The debates likely to be generated in this climate may well promote further research into mental and social health at work, as well as a deeper knowledge of more familiar areas, such as accident prevention and the toxicity of materials.

12.7   Noise

The most encouraging prospects for countering the insidious and growing problem of noise are based on increasing awareness of the problem and developing the will to deal with it. A step forward was taken in 1978, when member countries of the Organization for Economic Cooperation and Development formulated proposals for future noise abatement policies. They recognized the importance of the control of noise at source and publicity of the performance of appliances in this respect, as part of a general plan to improve consciousness and education of the public. Emphasis was given to the development of progressively more stringent standards, with incentives for good performance and a system of compensation for the recipients of noise, where no other remedy existed. A need was identified for the harmonization of measurement methods and the adoption of uncomplicated standards and means of applying them.

Noise in industry can be controlled, in many instances, without unreasonable levels of expenditure, provided that management policy is committed to planned measures for improvement. Such a programme has been undertaken at a Swedish factory and reported in detail (Engstrom, 1981). Finance was allocated over a period of several years for the improvement of working conditions, including noise surveys, remedial works and follow-up monitoring. The report points out that the incentive to produce quiet machines is greatly promoted by purchasers demanding that they meet specified acoustic performance standards. The report quotes an 8 dB(A) reduction in noise emission from a machine, achieved at a cost representing only 0.5% of the initial price, demonstrating that improvements need not always be costly.

Cost remains a problem, however, in dealing with road traffic noise. If the present qualification for sound insulation of houses newly affected by traffic noise (see Chap. 9) were improved from L_{10} 18-hour 68 dB(A) to 64 dB(A), an estimated 50% increase in costs would result. The more satisfactory method of putting new roads into cuttings would be very much more expensive (Transport and Road Research Laboratory, 1980).

Improved legislation available to local authorities (Control of Pollution Act 1974) is proving valuable in dealing with industrial, neighbourhood and construction noise problems which cannot be resolved by informal means. In the rare cases where summary proceedings are an insufficient solution, injunctions under section 58(8) of the Control of Pollution Act, or section 222 of the Local Government Act 1972 may be sought against offenders. The provisions to establish Noise Abatement Zones have not been widely exercised, but were designed to counter the effects of gradually increasing levels of noise and may well find wider application as experience in their use grows.

Liaison between Planning and Environmental Health Officers is a vital factor in preventing the introduction of noisy activities into quiet areas, and the same can be said of land uses involving the emission of fumes, dust and odours. The emphasis here should be on prevention of problems, rather than the application of a cure *post facto*.

12.8   Health education

All that has gone before relates to the global or macroenvironment determined fundamentally by the place where we live and the activities of the society of which we are a part. Within this, however, is the particular and personal environment which each individual creates for himself or herself, determined by that persons way of life — the microenvironment. Earlier chapters have shown how an important element of the ill-health which occurs in modern times is engendered by these much more personal aspects of activity. Such matters as preferences in eating and drinking, consumption of tobacco, alcohol or drugs, occupation, leisure pursuits, exercise, the amount of rest taken, and personal hygiene, are all important in influencing bodily health. So are concepts and beliefs about the ways in which people should act and interact, and the origins of disease, indeed the whole cultural pattern of existence. As the macroenvironment comes increasingly under legislative control, so those diseases related to bad sanitation and domestic pollution, such as infectious diseases, tend to disappear from the scene. Instead, those diseases related to the microenvironment become increasingly important.

Epidemiological research into such important causes of illness and premature mortality as coronary heart disease and lung cancer have shown that the microenvironment plays a vital part in their causation, and the reader of earlier chapters will have gleaned information about many other conditions in which personal habits and behaviour play a part. In such cases, it is only by influencing individual behaviour and ideas that the environmental causes of disease will be modified. Already, diseases which have their roots largely in the microenvironment place a heavy burden on the national economy; expensive treatments are devised in order to reverse the effects of conditions which, in theory at least, are susceptible to a fair amount of primary prevention which would be very much less costly.

However, it is not a simple matter to change the ways in which people behave. Cultural and social influences are strong, habits become ingrained and even addictive, concepts are passed from one generation to the next both by word of mouth and by example. The theoretical answer to this problem is to supply information about the influences which personal behaviour will have on personal health to the population at large, and to expect that they will then eschew habits and practices which lead to a greater risk of ill-health. In practice this does not occur, or, if it does, the process is painfully slow and usually only takes part in some sections of the community.

Nevertheless, the objective of health education is to influence personal behaviour and habits in such a way as to reduce influences which are damaging, and to promote the concept of positive health. The government is well aware of the ever-increasing importance of the microenvironment in the battle for improved health, and has given its blessing to this approach by creating the Health Education Council, and by issuing a number of informative publications of its own, including the pamphlet *Prevention and Health: Everybody's Business* (see p. 197). The Health Education Council was set up in 1969 when it supplanted the former Central Council for Health Education. Under the initial directorship of Mr Alistair MacKie, and recently of Professor Keith Taylor, and the guidance of some 27 members selected for their interest and expertise in health education, all appointed by the Secretary of State, the Council has developed a large number of initiatives. Many of the members are professionals in the health, education or social services; the main source of income of the organization is the national exchequer, and, in 1980, it spent over five million pounds. The functions of the Council, as summarized in its annual reports, are given in Table 12.3. Close attention is paid to all those facets of human behaviour which are recognized as promoting ill-health, and it is constantly working to reduce the toll of premature death which results. Various campaigns on self care, perinatal problems, smoking, alcoholism, and the use of health services are mounted by the Council on a nationwide basis, or sometimes in selected localities. Health education in schools is promoted, assistance on topics and materials is given to the teaching profession. Adult education is stimulated through contacts with adult education programmes run by local authorities and even through the Open University. The Council publishes and distributes posters and leaflets, and from time to time takes up advertising space in newspapers, magazines, on television and in the cinema. It publishes a quarterly journal, the *Health Education Journal*, aimed mainly at the professions engaged in health education, and containing reports of campaigns and discussion articles about health education technique. A

Table 12.3   Functions of the Health Education Council in the United Kingdom, as summarized in its annual reports. (Reproduced by permission of the Health Education Council.)

---

(1)   To advise on priorities for health education on the basis of the best information and evidence available.

(2)   To advise and carry out national campaigns, and local or regional campaigns in cooperation with Regional and Area Health Authorities and local authorities as appropriate.

(3)   To produce information and publicity material in support of national and local campaigns and of such other activities as the Council may undertake; and to make such material available to Area Health Authorities, local authorities and voluntary and other appropriate bodies.

(4)   To undertake or sponsor research and surveys designed to ensure that reliable and up-to-date information and statistics are available on which to base the campaigns and other activities of the Council.

(5)   To seek advice and to review relevant medical, epidemiological, sociological, psychological and other information available and, as necessary, to undertake or sponsor research and surveys designed to obtain such information to assist the Council in its determination or priorities and in the measurement of the effectiveness of the results of its national and experimental campaigns.

(6)   To act as the national centre of expertize and knowledge in all aspects of health education, so that advice is available at all times to Area Health Authorities and others engaged in health education; and, with the agreement of National Health Service and local authorities, educational and voluntary bodies, to coordinate health education activities where appropriate.

(7)   To encourage and promote training in health education work; and to provide to other bodies advice and guidance on the organization and content of courses of training, together with such practical help as may seem appropriate and within the resources of the Council.

(8)   To cooperate with local education authorities, educational establishments and the Schools Council in the development of health education in schools, colleges and polytechnics.

(9)   To maintain contact with national voluntary bodies engaged in particular aspects of health education work; and to give aid and advice to such bodies as appropriate and to the extent that the resources of the Council permit.

(10)   To publish material of interest and value to those engaged in health education.

---

central library and resource centre is maintained, at which exhibitions are staged and books and audio-visual aids are available.

This centrally based, and nationally orientated, organization is supplemented by local health education departments run by local health authorities. These are health education departments which heretofore have been under the control of the Area Health Authorities. With the recent reorganization of the health service these local health education offices will become directly responsible to the new District Health Authorities. Locally based health education officers have the responsibility of promoting and assisting on-going efforts at health education in their own localities, many have resource centres similar to that in London, and make materials and advice available to, for instance, local teachers, lecturers, health visitors and doctors. Local authorities are also taking an increasing interest in health education with respect to such matters as road safety and safety in the home, and through their public protection committees, appoint officers with specific responsibilities in these matters.

The Government publication *Prevention and Health: Everybody's Business* was prepared jointly by the Health Departments of Great Britain and Northern Ireland. After tracing the history of health over the previous century, and highlighting the remarkable decline of infectious diseases as a cause of mortality, the booklet turns its attention to current and future problems relating to ill-health in the nation. It points out the present day importance of heart disease, cancer and stroke as causes of death, and discusses aspects of human behaviour such as smoking, alcohol consumption, the mis-use of drugs, the use of leisure, and changes in views and con-cepts about human sexuality. The booklet then goes on to consider in some depth the potential scope for and practicalities of prevention. The book was intended to act as an initiator, encouraging widespread discussion about the issues involved, and ends by exhorting all those in the health education business to carry the work forward, developing local initiatives wherever possible. Clearly this was, and is, a major source of guidance to all those involved, from the Health Education Council downward, and set the seal of governmental approval on expenditure on health education directed along the lines which it proposed.

12.9   Finale

This book has examined in considerable detail the ways in which environment in-fluences human health and well-being. It has been shown repeatedly that, although natural factors determine the fundamental characteristics of the environment, the influences which human activity brings to bear upon it are extensive and of great significance. Humans have evolved in the natural environment and, over the ages, have adapted in such a way as to be the relatively efficient living organisms that they are today, but the sudden and dramatic changes which humans are now capable of inducing, ironically because of their advanced state of intellectual development, are too severe and too rapid to permit that kind of adaptation. By virtue of human intelligence, inquisitiveness, ability to communicate and to accumulate and integrate the information gained, by virtue of their ability to create and utilize tools and machinery and to mobilize large quantities of energy, humans have become a powerful agent of environmental change. Furthermore, the human race has increased vastly in numbers in recent centuries. One result has been the release of quantities of materials into the environment which is at risk of becoming overloaded and unable to recycle organic materials quickly enough. Some man-made materials cannot be recycled and can only accumulate. Such occurrences may bring unforeseen consequences in their train, or, even if they are foreseeable, it is difficult to bring about changes in practice which will safeguard the environment. Unfortunately humans tend to be inherently selfish; even when they can see poten-tial harm to the environment, and indirectly perhaps to themselves, they may not always easily be dissuaded from continuing, either through self-interest or just because of apathy. Education is obviously important, supported by good quality research, but equally important is the motivation to act upon it.

The extreme example of our power to damage our own environment is the current nuclear arms race between nations. The understanding which has been acquired of the power potential of nuclear fission is a scientific and technological advance which, at one and the same time, promises large supplies of energy which will be available when our stocks of fossil fuels have been used up, and threatens global catastrophe of unprecedented proportions if the new knowledge is mis-used. There are many less dramatic examples which have been quoted in previous pages, such as lead in petrol, freons in aerosols, accumulating pesticides and insecticides, or just the everyday pollution of the atmosphere generated by the burning of fossil fuels both in industry and in the home. Increasingly important is our maltreatment of our own bodies by deliberately inhaling smoke or living in unhygienic or even insanitary ways, eating inappropriate or frankly bad diets, and so on.

Both in terms of the macroenvironment and of the microenvironment, humans themselves hold the key to health and prosperity. They can change their environment for the better or the worse, depending upon the actions taken. First must come understanding and acceptance of relationships between environmental factors and health as have been outlined in this book, which, if it conveys no other message, demonstrates clearly that our future health is very largely in our own hands.

References

Anderson, J.M. (1981). *Ecology for Environmental Sciences: Biosphere, Ecosystems and Man*. Edward Arnold, London.

Avon, Gloucestershire and Somerset Environmental Monitoring Committee. Statement on Metals in Air, Indoor Firing Ranges. *The Rifleman*. Oct. 1979, pp. 8/33.

Barrington, E.J.W. (1980). *Environmental Biology*. Edward Arnold, London.

Beral, V. (1974). Cancer of the cervix: a sexually transmitted infection? *Lancet*, (i), 1037.

Bothwell, P.W. (1965). *A New Look at Preventative Medicine*. Pitman Medical Publishing Company.

Bowerman, J.M. (1979). *The CEGB and Nuclear Power. Questions and Answers*. Central Electricity Generating Board, London.

Bronte-Stewart, B., Keys, A., Brock, J.F., Moodie, A.D., Antonis, A. and Keys, M.H. (1955). *Lancet*, (ii), 1105.

Bruel and Kjaer. *Sound Measurement and Analysis*. Bruel and Kjaer, DK 2850, Naerum, Denmark.

Building Research Establishment. *BRE News, No. 53*, Spring 1981.

Burman, S. (Ed.) (1977). *Accidents in the Home*. Croom Helm, London.

Burns, W. (1973). *Noise and Man*, 2nd edition. William Clowes and Sons Ltd.

Cartier, P. (1952). Discussion following paper on 'Survey of some current British and European studies of occupational tumor problems' by W.E. Smith. *Archives of Industrial Hygiene*, 5, 262.

Chanlett, E.T. (1973). *Environmental Protection*. McGraw Hill.

Colley, J.R.T., Douglas, J.W.B. and Reid, D.D. (1973). Respiratory disease in young adults: influence of early childhood lower respiratory tract illness, social class, air pollution, and smoking. *British Medical Journal*, 3, 195.

Committee on the Problem of Noise (1963, reprinted 1973). Final Report, Cmnd 2065, H.M.S.O.

Conservation Society Working Party (1980). *Lead or Health*. The Conservation Society, 68 Dora Road, London SW19.

Davies, F.G. (1977). *Clay's Handbook of Environmental Health*, 14th edition. K.K. Lewis and Co. Ltd, London.

Department of the Environment, Welsh Office (1976). *Calculation of Road Traffic Noise*, 2nd impression. H.M.S.O.

Department of Health and Social Security (1980). *Lead and Health*. H.M.S.O.

Department of Health and Social Security (1981). *Health Trends*. H.M.S.O.

Doll, R. (1955). Mortality from lung cancer in asbestos workers. *British Journal of Industrial Medicine*. 12, 811.

Doll, R. (1967). *Prevention of Cancer, Pointers from Epidemiology*. Nuffield Provincial Hospitals Trust, London.

Duffus, J.H. (1980). *Environmental Toxicology*. Edward Arnold, London.

Engstrom, E. (1981) Systematic Noise Reduction Programme at Volvo BM, Eskilstuna. *Noise and Vibration Control Worldwide,* April, 97–100. Trade and Technical Press Ltd, East Molesey, Surrey.

Enos, W.F., Holmes, R.H. and Beyer, J. (1953). Coronary disease among United States soldiers killed in Korea. *Journal of the American Medical Association,* **152**, 1090.

Fairbairn, A.S. and Reid, D.D. (1958). Air pollution and other local factors in respiratory disease. *British Journal of Preventative and Social Medicine,* **12**, 94.

Fiennes, R. (1978). *The Environment of Man.* Croom Helm, London.

Haenszel, W. and Hillhouse, M. (1959). Uterine cancer morbidity in New York City and its relation to the pattern of regional variation within the United States. *Journal of the National Cancer Institute,* **22**, 1157.

Harlap, S. and Davies, A.M. (1974). Infant admissions to hospital and maternal smoking. *Lancet,* (i), 529.

Hawker, L.E. and Linton, A.H. (Eds) (1979). *Microorganisms. Function, Form and Environment,* 2nd edition. Edward Arnold, London.

Health Education Council (1976). *Prevention and Health: Everybody's Business.* H.M.S.O.

Hird, J.F.B. (1966). Planning for a new community. *Journal of the College of General Practitioners,* 12, Supplement 1.

Hobbs, B.C. and Gilbert, R.J. (1978). *Food Poisoning and Food Hygiene,* 4th edition. Edward Arnold, London.

Hochman, A., Ratzkowski, E. and Schreiber, H. (1955). Incidence of carcinoma of the cervix in Jewish women in Israel. *British Journal of Cancer,* **9**, 358.

Howe, G. Melvyn (Ed.) (1970). *National Atlas of Disease Mortality in the United Kingdom.* Thomas Nelson and Sons Ltd.

Hunter, D. (1981). *Diseases of Occupations.* English Universities Press.

International Labour Office (1976). *Occupational Health and Safety,* 5th impression. International Labour Office, Geneva.

Kinnersley, P. (1973). *The Hazards of Work; How to Fight Them.* Pluto Press.

McDonald, D.W. (1980). *Rabies and Wildlife.* Oxford University Press, Oxford.

McDonald, N. and Doyle, M. (1981). *The Stresses of Work.* Thomas Nelson and Sons Ltd.

McKeown, T. (1979). *The Role of Medicine: Dream, Mirage, or Nemesis?* Blackwell Scientific Publications, Oxford.

Mattingley, P.F. (1969). *The Biology of Mosquito borne Disease.* George Allen and Unwin Ltd.

Morris, J.N., Heady, J.A., Raffle, P.A.B., Roberts, C.G. and Parks, J.W. (1953). Coronary heart disease and physical activity of work. *Lancet,* (ii), 1053.

Murray, A. J. (1979). *Aquatic Environment Monitoring Report No. 2.* Ministry of Agriculture Fisheries and Food Directorate of Food and Fisheries Research, Lowestoft.

Newhouse, M.L. and Thompson, H. (1965). Mesothelioma of pleura and peritoneum following exposure to asbestos in the London area. *British Journal of Industrial Medicine,* **22**, 261.

Office of Population Censuses and Surveys (OPCS).
   (1974) Morbidity Statistics from General Practice. *Studies on Medical and Population Subjects No. 26.* H.M.S.O.
   (1978). *Occupational Mortality.* Decennial Supplement. 1970–72. England and Wales. H.M.S.O.

Palmer, K.N. (1954). The role of smoking in bronchitis. *British Medical Journal,* (i), 1473.

Ranson, R.P. (1979). The relationship between health and housing. *Environmental Health,* October, 227–9.

Rawls, W.E., Tompkins, W.A.F., Figuerora, M.E. and Melnick, J.C. (1968). Herpesvirus Type 2: Association with carcinoma of the cervix. *Science*, **161**, 1255.

Roberts, B.F. (1980). Food Hygiene — Quantifying the Risks. *Environmental Health*, November, 243–6.

Rous, P. (1911). A sarcoma of the fowl transmissable by an agent separable from the tumor cells. *Journal of Experimental Medicine*, **13**, 397.

Royal College of Physicians
(1962). *Smoking and Health*. Pitman, London.
(1971). *Smoking and Health Now*. Pitman, London.
(1977). *Smoking or Health*. Pitman, London.

Royal Commission on Environmental Pollution (1976). *Sixth Report — Nuclear Power and the Environment*.

Royal Commission on Environmental Pollution (1984). *Tenth Report — Tackling Pollution — Experience and Prospects*.

Sax, N.I. (1979). *Dangerous Prospects of Industrial Materials*. Van Nostrand Reinhold.

Scottish Council for Single Homeless (1981). *Think Single*.

Selikoff, I.J. *et al.* (1964). Asbestos exposure and neoplasia. *Journal of the American Medical Association*, **188**, 22.

Slack, J. and Evans, K. A. (1966). The increased risk of death from ischaemic heart disease in first degree relatives of 121 men and 96 women with ischaemic heart disease. *Journal of Medical Genetics*, **3**, 239.

Stocks, P. and Davies, R.I. (1964). Zinc and copper content of soils associated with the incidence of cancer of the stomach and other organs. *British Journal of Cancer*, **18**, 14.

Tobacco Research Council (1976). *Statistics of Smoking in the United Kingdom*. Research Paper 1. 7th edition.

Topley, C.C.W. and Wilson, G.S. (1975). *Principles of Bacteriology, Virology and Immunity*, 6th edition. Wilson, G.S. and Miles, A.A. (Eds). Edward Arnold, London.

Townsend, P. (1979). *Poverty in the United Kingdom*. Penguin.

Townsend, P. and Davidson, N. (Eds). (1982). *Inequalities in Health (The Black Report)*. Penguin.

Transport and Road Research Laboratory
(1974). Report No. 624.
(1980). Supplementary Report 475.

Wagner, J.C., Slegg, C.A. and Marchand, P. (1960). Diffuse pleural mesothelioma and asbestos exposure in the North Western Cape Province. *British Journal of Industrial Medicine*, **17**, 260.

Yudkin, J. (1964). Dietary fat and dietary sugar in relation to ischaemic heart disease and diabetes. *Lancet*, (ii), 4.

Index

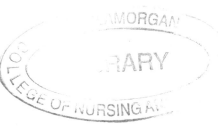

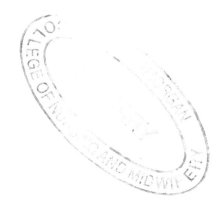